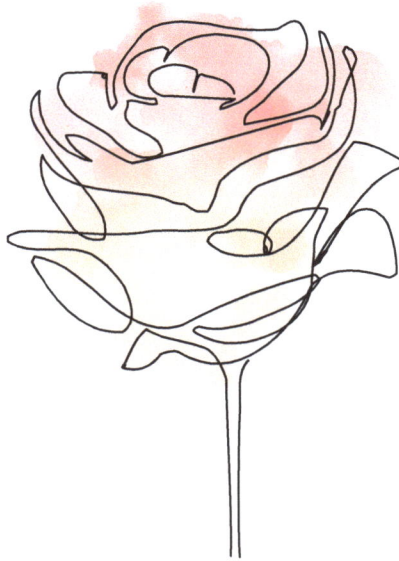

*To the boy who handed me a cardboard box*
*within which lay a piece of gold:*
*the gold is still intact.*

*To my godparents, May and Ken Copp.*
*Thank you.*

While books are designed for general use, please consider the following safety precautions: Ensure that the content of this book is appropriate for the intended age group. Keep this product out of reach of young children unless specifically designed for their age group. Supervision is recommended for children under 3 years of age due to potential risks such as small detachable elements, sharp corners, or the possibility of paper cuts. Avoid exposure to fire, heat sources, or water to maintain product integrity and prevent hazards.

**EU Conformity Declaration**

This product complies with the following safety regulations and standards to ensure consumer safety and product quality: Regulation (EU) 2023/988 of the European Parliament and of the Council on General Product Safety (GPSR): The Consumer Product Safety Improvement Act (CPSIA), Section 101. The Californian Safe drinking water and toxic enforcement act. (Proposition 65) EN71-Part 1: Mechanical and Physical Properties EN71-Part 2: Flammability EN71-Part 3 Migration of certain elements.

Produced by Softwood Books

EU Responsible person: Maddy Glenn
Office 2, Wharfside House, Prentice Road, Stowmarket, Suffolk, IP14 1RD
www.softwoodbooks.com
hello@softwoodbooks.com

EU Rep:
Authorised Rep Compliance Ltd.,
Ground Floor, 71 Lower Baggot Street, Dublin, D02 P593, Ireland
www.arccompliance.com
info@arccompliance.com

Published by **Heather Dawn Godfrey**
Text © **Heather Dawn Godfrey**
Cover design & layout by **www.coastline.agency**

**ISBN: 978-1-0685013-0-2 (Print)**
ISBN: 978-1- 0685013-1-9 (eBook)

**Other publications by Heather Dawn Godfrey**

Healing with Essential Oils:
*The Antiviral, Restorative, and Life-Enhancing Properties of 58 Plants.*

Essential Oils for the Whole Body:
*The Dynamics of Topical Application and Absorption*

Essential Oils for Mindfulness and Meditation:
*Relax. Replenish. Rejuvenate*

Visit Heather Dawn Godfrey's website:
**www.aromantique.co.uk**

# ESSENTIAL OILS
## *to*
# EASE ANXIETY

## ENDORSEMENTS

*In these challenging times where many people suffer from anxiety and stress, this book stands as a beacon of hope and resilience, offering a scientifically grounded and empathetic approach to mental wellbeing. The author skilfully combines research with practical applications, demonstrating the significant physiological and psychological benefits of essential oils on the brain, central nervous system, immune system, and endocrine system. Through the author's authentic narratives of personal loss and vulnerability, the book guides readers towards reclaiming control and balance. Supported by evidence, it explores how these natural remedies can alleviate symptoms of anxiety, depression, insomnia, and grief. This work is an invaluable resource for practitioners and individuals seeking evidence-based methods to enhance overall wellbeing and resilience, reminding us of our capacity for growth and transformation.*

**Emma-Jane Loveridge**
Health Expert and Author

*This book is an illuminating exploration of aromatherapy!
I felt as though I'd been invited into a realm where the essence of
nature meets the intricate workings of our mind, body, and spirit.
Heather is clearly an alchemist and has a profound understanding of
the power of essential oils and the transformative potential they hold
within every drop.*

*I learnt how essential oils transcend mere fragrances to become potent
allies in our quest for holistic well-being. Drawing from ancient
traditions and modern science alike, she intricately weaves together
the threads of history, spirituality, and healing to create a tapestry of
wisdom that resonates deeply with the soul. This is a book to remind
us that within the embrace of essential oils, we can find solace,
healing and a deeper sense of wholeness.*

**Janey Lee Grace**
Author and Broadcaster

*Heather's book is a treasure trove of information and wisdom which
links essential oils to every aspect of life. It is a timely reminder of
the remedies available within the natural world which have served
humanity long before the advent of big pharma.*

**Ian Mouland**
Director Mouland Mann
(Specialist Search and Merger Consultancy)

# Rhiannon Lewis

In 2022, the World Health Organization's report "World Mental Health Report: Transforming Mental Health for All" highlighted the growing global need for improved care strategies in the area of mental health – a sector that is typically underfunded and currently inadequate to meet the acute and long-term needs of those suffering. What is more, with one in eight people living with a mental health disorder (thirteen per cent of the global population) and with just two per cent of health expenditure allocated to mental healthcare, this global public health burden is on track to further increase.

The growing shift towards integrative personalised care is especially important for those with depression and associated anxiety disorders. Depression is the leading cause of disability around the world yet we now know that more than thirty per cent of those with a major depressive disorder do not respond to first line standardised 'one-size fits all' treatment. Similarly, for those with generalised anxiety disorder, approximately fifty per cent do not respond to first line care. As the efficacy gaps in the mental health arena are acknowledged and with increasing numbers of young people diagnosed with anxiety and depression, identifying and implementing complementary and safe strategies to support traditional medical care thereby reducing polypharmacy and improving the impact of first line treatment are increasingly welcomed. Tailoring treatment to individual needs is paramount.

What is more, in this anxiogenic age where there is a sense of disconnection, isolation and an increasing fear of the future coupled with loss of choice and autonomy, there is value in turning towards the natural world and the rhythmicity of seasons. Many express a hunger to return to a simpler and more natural world where the 'wheel that turns' is predictable, familiar, comforting and soothing. Nature has the capacity to prime positive emotions and reduce negative affect. This human-nature connection has an undeniable emotional dimension. Advocates of biophilia, as publicised by the evolutionary biologist Edward O. Wilson since the 1980's would argue that we possess an innate, human instinct to connect with the natural world.

When one is in a state of hyper or hypo arousal, when the outside world seems too difficult, too strange or too dangerous to navigate, the power of scent, and essential oils are uniquely placed to immediately bring comfort, familiarity and empowerment. With simple self-care strategies to enhance wellbeing and to provide a space for breath and for calm, essential oils provide the opportunity to bring the natural world directly to the brain. With a single breath, the power of aroma can transport the person to safety, calm and enhanced balance. The olfactory sense provides the space to pause, rebalance, reconnect, uplift and restore perspective.

Over the recent ten years, there has been a growing emphasis in the mental health profession on the importance of encouraging a healthy lifestyle alongside medical care. This is coupled with the recognition of the value of promoting self-care, resilience and empowerment as safe, effective and cost-effective approaches to be integrated into individualised treatment for depression and associated anxiety disorders. Integration is indeed the key to success and aromatherapy beautifully and safely complements standard psychiatric care practices.

This text by Heather Dawn Godfrey is therefore very timely. Heather is well placed to write on this topic. As with her previous publications, through her well researched information and easily accessible writing style, she guides and enables the general reader to take positive, pragmatic, doable steps towards improving their own mental health. Through her longstanding experience as therapist, educator and award-winning author, Heather provides simple tools and strategies for priming and maintaining an inner locus of balance and control.

*Rhiannon is editor of the International Journal of Clinical Aromatherapy and a clinical aromatherapy practitioner with over thirty years of professional experience. She also organises and hosts international aromatherapy related conferences, trade shows and events (for example, Botanica conference and trade show for clinical aromatherapy and phytotherapy, and the Essence of Clinical Aromatherapy International Seminar) and is a Director of the International Clinical Aromatherapy Network (ICAN) learning and networking resource.*

# ACKNOWLEDGEMENTS

I have discovered and learned so much over the decades, through study and experiential practice. However, the adage, 'the more you learn the less you know', is very true; there will always remain more to explore and discover. In truth, I realise, I am a perpetual student on an ever-evolving and revealing journey.

As always, I acknowledge that while writing is an insular process requiring my full attention, the outcome is never fully achieved without the support, thoughtfulness and kindness of others. I am grateful for the shared wisdom, insight and feedback generously shared. I am also grateful to other authors, teachers and researchers who contribute to the universal pool of knowledge and information; like the elephant and the blind men, each touch and hold fragments of truth that weave the bigger picture.

Briefly, but not exclusively, I especially wish to thank
**Sophie Olszowski, Vicky Dixon, Emma-Jane Loveridge, Ian Mouland, Sue Stone, Janey Lee Grace, Pamela Allsop,** and my brother
**Stephen Godfrey,** for their ongoing support and
belief in my endeavours.

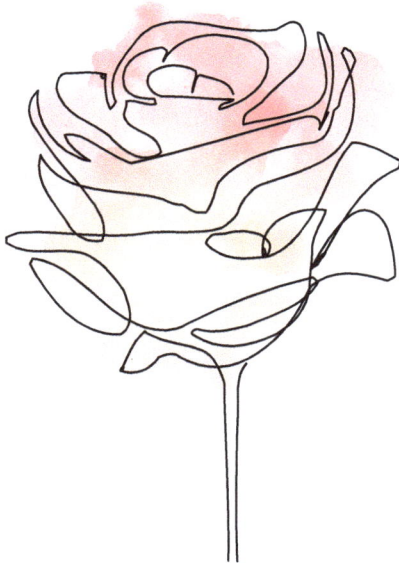

# CONTENTS

# CONTENTS

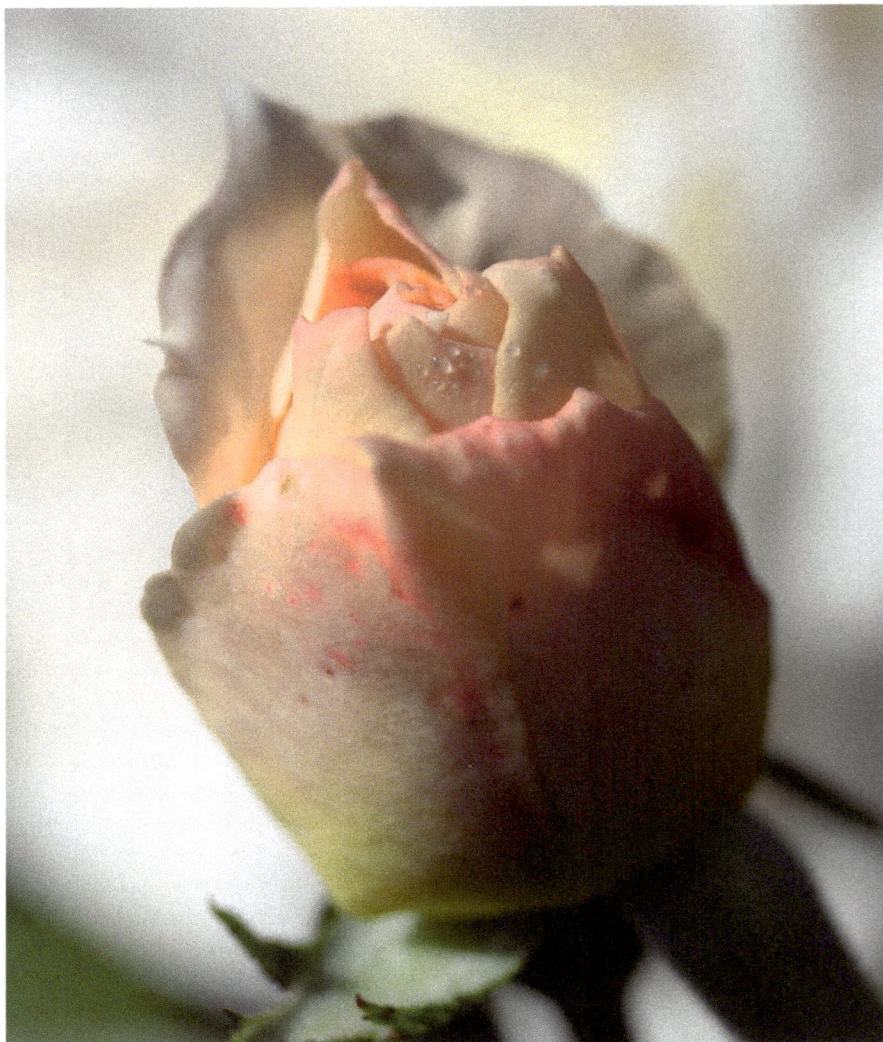

# Anxiety in context

It is impossible to be alive at the moment without being aware of the 'times' we are travelling through, or to remain unaffected by the impact or implication this awareness has on our existential sense of safety and security. I do not wish or intend to be yet another harbinger of doom and gloom, but it feels incongruent not to acknowledge this state of 'current affairs' when discussing or bringing the subject of anxiety, or depression, into the foreground. Indeed, when set against this backdrop the subject of essential oils, meditation or relaxation, may seem mute or benign, even absurdly trivial.

James Redfield, in his Celestine Prophecy book series, acknowledges the burgeoning 'end time' polarity between 'positive' and 'negative', darkness and light; one vying to destructively over-power, the other simply expanding into the higher realms of grace and love; an unfolding Armageddon-like spiritual battle between evil and good. Yet, as Redfield's heroes eventually discover, the war is already won; rising levels of consciousness dissolve the battle-cry. Simply, darkness cannot exist in the presence of light; dis-spelled by light, darkness doesn't disappear, it doesn't go anywhere, it simply does not exist. The desperate vying for power is merely the despairing, all-be-it horrific, last throes of darkness as the sun dawns above the horizon. But this is a ridiculously naive and over-simplified notion, I am repeatedly told. Yet, is it? Am I naïve? I am almost seventy years old. I have experienced pain, despair, loss, 'dark nights of the soul'. I absolutely realise that my pain is not your pain, my story is not your story, but are we really so different? I have experienced and witnessed the hand of darkness; sometimes a gentle insidious whispered touch, sometimes a brutal swipe, sometimes creeping in the shadows like a stalking predator.

Then, there are those things that happen in life because they are part of the 'journey'; relationship breakups, losing a job or promotion, a bad rainy season that beats sodden crops into the ground, birth and death, marriage and divorce, and the things that you cannot control due to the decisions, actions and non-actions of others. My father passed away suddenly nearly thirty years ago. No warning, no expectation. I was devasted, shocked, deeply heart broken, completely unprepared; no chance to say 'goodbye', no farewell hug or chance to voice unspoken words, my grief was all consuming. My father was my childhood rock. We spent hours talking with each other when I was a young teenager, just me and him, about the 'things of life'. I loved our conversations. He guided my moral compass. I valued his insight and openness (more now than I realised at the time). He had just retired, my children were grown, here was my chance to sit and mull over the things of life with him again. The bottle of lavender I dug from the bottom of my bag didn't quell my anguish, dry my tears, remove the pain from my heart, but somehow, in the midst of my despair, I felt unexplainably soothed and comforted by its scent; it didn't change anything, I still had to walk through my grief, but the broken jagged edge of my despair subtly softened – I could cope.

In truth, the battle and the peace lie within each of us; in every choice, in every decision we make, in every action and non-action, in our voice and in our silence, we influence the 'picture'. Honesty, with self and others, is always the 'best foot forward'; responsibility, integrity, respect and honour, pave the hero's path; do no harm, a common law; love, a spiritual truth; pain and suffering, wings unfurling. I hear my father's words echo in my musing. We are paradoxically interdependent autonomous individuals; we are sovereign beings gifted with incredible potential. In spite of our trials and tribulations, our capacity to heal and thrive is boundless; we are alchemists, if we so choose to be. While I create remedies, all healing, ultimately, comes from within.

'End times' or not, this book aims to support you maintain your personal locus of control in terms of managing and nurturing health and wellbeing. Essential oils instigate significant physiological influence on the brain and central nervous system, the immune system and micro-biome, the endocrine system, and also, poignantly, they exhibit significant psycho-emotional-spiritual qualities that may ground, balance and uplift mood, improve memory and recall, and thus generally support mental health; perfect travelling companions.  Gifts of nature, essential oils (resins and herbs) feature in many traditional ancient, and modern, medicinal and spiritual canons, including the Bible, and other scriptures.  As you will discover in the following pages, essential oils, alongside other related remedial strategies and ancient wisdoms (for there is no such thing as one cure-all strategy), can ease the symptoms of anxiety (and accompanying co-morbidities, such as depression, insomnia, fear and grief), potentially subtly softening the broken jagged edges, while healing takes place.

For ease of reading and information retrieval, the following content is divided into two sections and twenty-three short chapters.  Section One, Walking with Anxiety, explores what anxiety is, it's cause and consequence and ways to determine, manage and alleviate symptoms.  Section Two, Applying Essential Oils, explains the multiple dynamical properties and qualities of essential oils and identifies remedial psycho-emotional-spiritual indications for sixty individual essential oils, including their associated traditional energetic and subtle elements, that will assist you to hone and individualise selection of the most pertinent oil, or oils, in accord with your specific need or requirement.

SECTION ONE:

# Walking with Anxiety

*This section explores the cause and consequence of anxiety and ways to determine, manage and alleviate symptoms.*

## 1. What is Anxiety?

Anxiety is both a friend and a curse.

As a friend, anxiety protects and warns us when something is 'out of sync'. It fuels vigilance and triggers a neurological response that prepares the body for expedient action. A valuable indicator of imminent danger or threat, a signal light. Heads-up, we are able to appropriately respond. Thank you.

Unattended, anxiety lingers like an unwelcome guest, beckoning fear and dread for company; terrifying bedfellows. Chest heavy, throat tight, there's no room left to breathe. A strangling, suffocating spell that castes its victim into the shadows of a dark void; unearthed, free-floating, petrified. Racing heart, sweating, cold, pale and weak, trembling debilitation smothers resolve, panic attacks the last bastion.

Not a flight of fancy. I have stood, terrified, on this earthless ground, like a stringless puppet; a state I would not wish on my worst enemy - and yet I know I am not alone in experiencing its grip. The first time I experienced the all-consuming anxiety I felt I had been thrust into hell, a dark, suffocating, terrifying, bottomless pit. The second time, although nonetheless just as consuming and terrifying, I at least knew the nightmare would, eventually, pass. But, while the experience does pass, its imprint never completely leaves, and I have learned to walk beside this highly sensitive trait, to distinguish between natural, useful anxiety, and 'saturation' anxiety, which arrives, often insidiously, when I take on too much, feel too much, absorb too much.

There can be numerous triggers, or causes, some obvious and some subtle; it may be many small things, it may be just one. When anxiety surges within me, I do not fight against this unwelcome guest, or try to dismiss or 'block it out' (which is impossible to do anyway). I have learned to acknowledge it as I might a friend, to travel alongside, observing, allowing it to reveal its message to me, to teach me, guide me. And if my anxiety begins to become overwhelming (for now, I recognise the warning signs well in advance) I relax and surrender, slow down, take life one moment, one situation, at a time; if necessary, I reduce my commitments; rest and nourish myself; reduce or eliminate my caffeine intake; seek the company of good friends; go for short walks and gratefully breathe with nature; find a good book to lose myself within, to distract my attention from my angst; apply grounding, balancing and uplifting essential oils to ease my angst and soothe my mood and emotion (as with the bottle of lavender, above). By acknowledging the signs as they arise, by slowing down and stepping back, I am able to differentiate, to identify the real culprit, to respond appropriately; turn myself away from the gates of hell.

But this is not always easy to do. I recognise there are times I also need support. That mutual support is imperative, vital (in all healing scenarios), as isolation, separation, and loneliness, are the hand maidens of mental and emotional, and ultimately physical, demise. We are, after all, gregarious social beings who thrive in good community and excel when we live congruently with ourselves, with each other, with nature, and with purpose, and nurture and support each other; united by our differences and likenesses in equal measure. Autonomous interdependent beings; a perpetual existential paradox.

This phenomenon is apparently true in nature too. Peter Wohlleben, German forester, film maker and author, in his fascinating book, *The Hidden Life of Trees* (2016), for example, describes how trees of the same species that grow locally to each other share life-sustaining nutrients via root connections and networks. *The trees, it seems,* Wohlleben explains (p 12 - 17), *are equalising differences between the strong and the weak, whoever has an abundance of sugar hands some over, whoever is running short gets some help, thus, ensuring that each tree can grow to the best that it can be - a bit like the way social security systems operate to ensure individual members of society don't fall too far behind.*

Similarly, Merlin Sheldrake, biologist and author, in his equally fascinating book, *Entangled Life: how fungi make our worlds, change our minds, and shape our futures* (2020 p 235), discusses in deliberating detail how connections between the roots of individual trees, and plants, are made possible by facilitating fungal mycorrhizal networks that spread underground; a sort of deal is struck whereby nutrients and information are exchanged to the mutual benefit of all parties (trees, plants and fungi). Just like human relationships, this bio-ecological interaction involves negotiated trade-offs and compromises, Sheldrake explains, sometimes referred to as a form of socialism (as above, and, no doubt, meant in its simplicist, or purest, non-political sense), a means by which the wealth of the forest can be redistributed and shared; younger trees are nourished by their fungal connections to older and larger mother trees, thus, creating and sustaining a mutually collaborative, synergistic environment.

Trees also communicate information via means of electrical signals relayed through nerve-like cells at the tips of the roots, and above ground through olfactory, visual and sound (vibrational resonance). Dr Zach Bush (2021), physician, educator and founder of Farmer's Footprint, refers to this process as a form of 'quorum sensing' (cell to cell information sharing), a phenomenon by which collaborating species are enabled to evolve (create or catalyse) mutually cooperative and beneficial hyper-intelligent systems.

When isolated from this network, lone saplings or trees do not fare well. Standing alone, they forego the protection afforded by this communal communicative interface and material exchange; they are less able to curtail microbial invasion, they do not recover well from damage, they do not grow to their full capacity or live as long as other, mutually supported trees. And this is where Wohlleben's, Sheldrake's and others, personified metaphors of nature share and shine light on a common truth; as social beings, we too tend to thrive in positive supportive company, we too similarly do not fare well in isolation from each other; our mental, emotional and physiological well-being depends on positive mutual support, communication, feedback and nourishment if we are to thrive and synergise to our full capacity, to stretch and grow.

## 2. What causes anxiety?

Triggers of anxiety are manifold.

Official diagnostic tools, however, are concise and simplified and generally divide anxiety into two, potentially overlaying, modes: *state* and *trait*. *State anxiety* is fleeting, does not last or linger, and is associated with a responsive temporary increase in sympathetic nervous system activity (fight or flight, for example), which disappears with the removal of the triggering stressor or perceived danger. *Trait anxiety* is described as an inherent aspect of who a person is, a predisposition of their personality and how they tend to respond to and process life events and potential stress-triggers and situations of high arousal; in this scenario, anxiety is easily activated but does not disappear easily when the trigger or stressor is removed or relieved. (Tan et al 2023; Zsido et al 2020; Speilberger 1983). Anxiety, however, is not simplistic; boundaries blur and overlap, the 'felt' experience can be both subtle and overwhelming, cause and response multifaceted.

In the first instance, at the more subtle end of this continuum, or spectrum, anxiety may manifest as a sense of foreboding, of discomfort, of feeling uneasy or incongruent. In this instance, we may experience feelings of anxiousness as if it is a warning light that something is not 'right'; for example, that 'gut feeling' that instantly alerts us to be vigilant, or signals when we are not being true to ourselves or are out of sync in some way. Perhaps we are not honouring our physical needs for rest and nourishment; perhaps we are spending too much time alone or, conversely, spending too much time without personal space and privacy; perhaps we have too little or too much to do; spend too much time over focused on one task or project, or 'over thinking'; take on too much responsibility; are in the wrong relationship or job.

At the other end of this continuum or spectrum, as described earlier, anxiety can be terrifying, paralysing, perhaps experienced as a sense of extreme panic or existential overwhelm or unexplained threat, or as feelings of disassociation or derealisation (that is, feeling disconnected from the world around you, or that the world is not real). Psychological, emotional and physical shock, horror, mental harm or abuse, obvious and insidious (one may be sudden, the other creeps up), can thrust us into a state of terror or extreme anxiety, or, seemingly conversely, into a state of defensive inertia or 'numbness'.

Feelings of anxiety can also arise in response to a sensitivity reaction to foods or chemicals, including certain medications, that we may consume or come into contact with. For example, a blood-sugar imbalance can instigate feelings of anxiousness, restlessness or unease, so can high blood pressure and other heart conditions. Culprits include:

- Caffeine, alcohol, sugary drinks, fruit juice and artificial sweeteners, and certain foods.

- Processed foods.

- Pharmaceutical drugs such as aspirin, ibuprofen, cortisone, Ritalin, betablockers, opiates, among others.

- Industrial metals and chemicals, such as lead (for example, found in paint, jewellery and drinking water), mercury (found in fish, dental fillings, pharmaceuticals, and batteries), toluene (found in paint thinners, nail polish, varnish and glues), ethanol (found in alcoholic drinks, pharmaceutical skin lotions, cosmetics and perfumes), and fluoride (found in synthetic fluoridated tap water, dental products, and mouth washes, and natural trace amounts found in foods such as bananas and avocados), among others.

• Physical imbalance or dis-ease: for example, gut microbiome imbalance, heart problems, diabetes, and hypoglycaemia.

Clearly, in some circumstances, a sense of foreboding or anxiousness actually is a 'heads up' or warning that 'something is not right'.

## 3. Anxiety and depression

Anxiety and depression are never far from each other, sometimes they even appear to snuggle up to each other, indistinguishably merging. Indeed, where anxiety goes, depression follows, and vice versa; although this is not always absolutely the case.   Matt Haig, for example, observes in his poignant book *Reasons to Stay Alive* (2016), that anxiety, more than depression, is triggered and exacerbated by life in the twenty first century. He eloquently and humorously (which instils a sense of optimism rather than despair) invites the reader to journey with him through the lens of his first-hand lived experience of being in these states.  In mapping the territory, describing the dark and light contours, the hidden depths and valleys, the mountain tops, of this undulating terrain, he reminds the reader that as lonely or frighteningly isolated they may feel tumbling into this landscape, they are not alone or alien, it is, indeed, a well-trodden path; that no matter how bleak or terrifying, there is always a pathway through, one step, one moment, at a time.

See the *Signs, Symptoms and Causes of Anxiety and Depression* chart in Appendix One.

## 4. Being highly sensitive

According to Elaine Aron, author of *The Highly Sensitive Person* (1999), fifteen to twenty-percent of the population are potentially highly sensitive; some estimate even higher, for example, up to thirty-percent (Dosari et al 2023).  Highly sensitive people (HSP's), Aron explains, are inclined to be more aware of the subtleties and nuances of their surroundings, are easily overwhelmed by sensory stimulation, feel emotionally saturated and tire very quickly, and often need to retreat to be alone and quiet, to gather their senses, feelings and thoughts.  Responses to over-arousal and fear often appear very similar to each other and one can easily be mistaken for the other in the throes of the moment; for example, our heart may be pounding from the sheer effort of processing extra stimulation.  Other similar symptoms, or expressions, Aron explains, include shaking hands, trembling, foggy thoughts, muscles tensing, stomach churning, hands or other parts of the body perspiring, and blushing (p 10).  As before, being aware of these similarities, and differentiating between sensitivity and anxiety, may arrest one from spilling into the other; over-arousal and feelings of overwhelm and saturation then do not insidiously slip on the additional garments of fear and panic.

(Dosari et al 2023; Farmer et al 2015; Aron 2004, 1999)

See the *Traits of the Highly Sensitive Person* chart in Appendix One.

## 5. Learning to live with anxiety

How we respond to life's challenges differs from one person to another; we all have different coping mechanisms, attitudes, and saturation points. Stress is one of many triggers that may tip the balance. Significantly, and similarly, Hans Seyle (1907-1982), founder of the stress theory (known also as the 'father of stress research'), identified two types of stress; *eu*-stress, which acts as a positive drive or motivator, and *dis*-stress, which can trigger a negative and potentially debilitating psycho-emotional (and consequently, a physiological) reaction that may ultimately lead to *dis*-ease (Tan and Yip 2018). The Oxford English Dictionary defines stress as *overwhelming pressure experienced by someone or something as a result of some adverse force or influence;* indeed, stress and pressure are terms that are sometimes referred to synonymously. Our response to stress, however, determines whether it is positive or negative to us, and whether it invites other 'guests' to the party.

It appears that through our attitude we possess the alchemy to transfigure metal into gold, if we so choose. Challenge, for example, invites us to leave our comfort zones, push our boundaries, and may instil many benefits such as, improved alertness, vigilance, performance, and an enhanced sense of quality of life. However, even positive pressure, or challenge, when relentless or excessive, loses its beneficial effect; in the instance of stress, balance tipped, *eu*-stress insidiously becomes *dis*-stress, pressure, once motivating and invigorating, then, if left unchecked, becomes destructive and harmful, and mental, emotional and physical health and wellbeing may consequently suffer.

Some stress-triggers or causes of anxiety, as previously established, are controllable and others are not, but in all cases, awareness of the cause and consequence of whatever the trigger may be (and there can be many small things) helps to peel back the layers, to differentiate between what is avoidable and what is not, what is a useful signalling mechanism, and what is destructive; thus, through this process of considered evaluation and elimination, the potential negative culprits are whittled down and appropriate remedial strategies can be more efficiently and effectively assigned. Sometimes, just being aware of a cause - the renewed perspective this may afford - is sufficient remedy.

There are numerous books that explore the causes and symptoms of anxiety and depression, and sensitivity too. Matt Haig, in *Reasons to Stay Alive* (2016 p 189), reminds us, however, that while our experience overlaps with other peoples, it is never exactly the same experience, and that while umbrella labels are useful descriptors, they do not begin to encapsulate the complex dynamics of the unique real-lived experience of the individual; there is no one-size-fits-all description nor one-size-fits-all remedy.

## 6. The cornerstones of wellbeing

We assist our flourishing when we acknowledge certain basic principles underpinning our daily living, for example:

- Eating fresh, nutritionally dense and balanced, and preferably, seasonal, organic food, and remaining sufficiently hydrated (drinking fresh water and eating fresh vegetables and fruits, which also contain water, as well as vital minerals and trace elements).

- Being outside and exposed to natural seasonal light, environmental elements, and nature.

- Exercise, movement and mobility.

- Meditation, prayer, and relaxation.

- Sufficient sleep (optimally, eight hours, commencing at least two hours before midnight, and absent electronic devices).

- Love, joy, friendship, community, work and sense of purpose, honesty with self and others.

(O'Neill 2024; Godfrey 2022 p.141; Heying and Weinstein 2021)

These principles are covered in more depth in my previous books, *Essential Oils for Mindfulness and Meditation,* and *Healing with Essential Oils.* However, to reiterate some key points here.

The way we eat, as well as the nutrient density and freshness of the food we consume, impact and influence how the body assimilates vital minerals and nutrients required to support metabolic processes; this, in turn, affects our health and feelings of wellbeing (mental, emotional, and physiological). Energy surrendered to us by this process fuels physiological activity, movement and motion, strength and resilience, also cognitive function and awareness (which includes mood, emotion, attitude, tolerance and clarity of thought). We share ancient cellular life-force memories and intelligence with plants; indeed, we are in vital dynamical, mutualistic and synergistic relationship, not only with each other, but also with our surrounding environment. (Heying and Wienstien 2022; Sayer Ji 2022, 2020; Wood 2021; Gagliano 2017).

Lack of and / or poor assimilation of vitamins, minerals and trace elements (which are potentiated by sunlight, water and oxygen – sunlight, for example, potentiates the production of vitamin D within the body, which supports our immune system, calcium homeostasis and bone metabolism) invariably results in physiological disharmony. Significantly, for example, lack of vitamin B1 (found in foods such as liver, milk, eggs, green leafy vegetables, molasses, and legumes) may lead to, or exacerbate, nervous disorders and physical symptoms, such as anxiety, low thyroid function, appetite loss, heart palpations, and feelings of fear, sensitivity to noise, irritability, confusion, loss of morale, and nervous exhaustion. Lack of vitamin B3, B5, B6 and B9 (found in kidney, eggs, avocado, carrots, molasses and dried fruit) may lead to, or exacerbate, feelings of irritability and depression. Lack of minerals, such as calcium (found in milk, cheese, walnuts, sesame and sunflower seeds, honey and molasses), potassium (found in citrus fruits, bananas, nuts, potatoes and green leafy vegetables), and iodine (found in sea salt, kelp and onions), may lead to or exacerbate feelings of nervousness. Insufficient vitamin D leads to fatigue (also myopia and poor bone density, and compromised immune function).

Dehydration (which occurs when we lose more fluid than we take in) may also lead to feelings of anxiety, agitation, even panic attacks (and other deleterious physiological consequences, such as, increased risk of heart attack or stroke, among other things).

Water within the body's cells is present in a liquid crystalline, plasma-like or structured state ($H^3O^2$) - the fourth phase of water, for example, 1. Ice, 2. EZ (exclusion zone or structured water), 3. Liquid, 4. Steam (Pollack 2016). Water accounts for about seventy percent of our cells total mass (without water our cells collapse and die). Our brain mass is composed of about seventy-five percent water, along with about sixty percent fat (insufficient intake of dietary saturated fats – animal fat and omega-3 and -6 fats and oils found in coconut, meat, fish, eggs, and walnuts, for example – is also linked with anxiety and depression). (Fado et al 2022; Larrieu 2018; Chang et al 2009; Bourre 2006) Water (in its liquid or vapour state) is perpetually excreted from our body; in our breath, sweat, urine, faeces, tears, blood and other bodily fluids. Water is a vital bodily component; indeed, our body cannot survive for more than three days without consuming replenishing fresh water, so feelings of anxiety and panic are clearly useful 'warning signs' if our 'well' is running low.

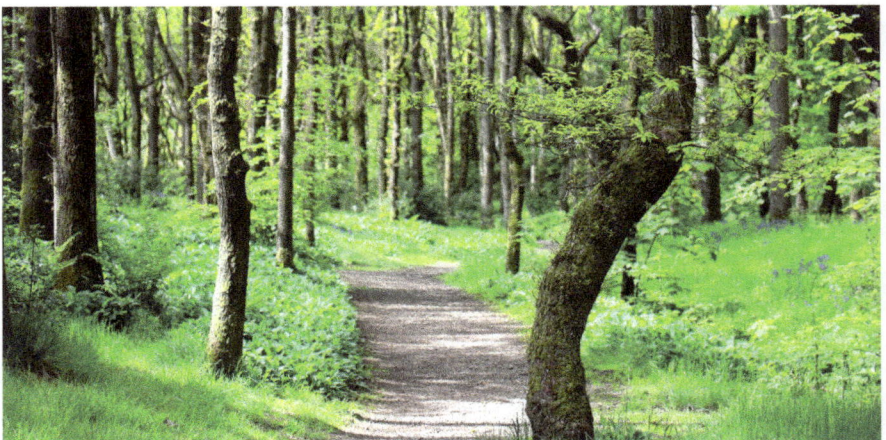

## 7. Indoors and outdoors

As Heying and Weinstein remind us in *A Hunter-Gather's Guide to the 21st Century* (2022), pre-industrial humans lived in communion with nature; in or near woods and forests, valleys, grassland, by rivers or seashores, with the sky above, soil beneath foot, feeling the elements, wind and rain, sensing the atmosphere, in tune with natural rhythms, light and dark, sunshine and storms, feast and famine; our instincts and senses acutely attuned to our environments.

Terms such as 'outdoors' and 'indoors', are modern phenomena. Our apparent advancement (technology, innovation, collaboration), it is true, brings many advantages (among other factors, the harshness of the elements, feast and famine, are tempered). But at what cost? So many of us (particularly in the West, unless you are a farmer, a forester, or such like) spend most our time 'inside', in unnatural square buildings in square rooms illuminated by artificial light, drenched in stagnant recycled atmospheres; we walk on concrete or speed about in closed vehicle bubbles; we spend time 'outside' on 'holiday' as if a luxury, we 'go for orchestrated walks' to offset our sedentary 'in doors' lifestyles.

'Environmental enrichment', a modern notion originally reserved for zoo animals living in caged captivity, now applies to humans too. Incongruent with our body's nature-al 'way of being' and our vital connection with our earthly environment, we are increasingly out-of-sync, out-of-sorts, out-of-wellness, our warning lights screaming (the promising and enticing glossy cover peeling at the edges); anxiety, depression, chronic illness, evidential witness of our disconnect.

Captured by our modern lifestyles, we seek positive ways to counterbalance this unhealthy trend, to restore natural equilibrium. As above, eating fresh, seasonal, natural food and drinking sufficient fresh water, is one step (Ji

2020).   Another, is seeking ways to return to being in a flow of motion and movement; exercise, dance, yoga, trekking 'off road', walking or simply standing barefoot in the grass, climbing the stairs instead of taking the lift, and so on (Mahindru et al 2023, Mikkelsen et al 2017, Oschman et al 2015, Chevalier 2015). Yet another, to reacquaint with stillness and silence, with doing 'nothing', with boredom, pondering, observation, contemplation, reflection, meditation and prayer (Peterson 2023, Rawat 2021, Tolle 2003). Also, being in communion, supporting, creating, loving, laughing, telling stories, breathing life into relationship, honouring our sovereignty and interdependence, our élan vital; appreciation and gratitude in motion.

## 8. Returning to the forest

This book aims to offer a tentative shoot, a root thread, one of many, that may connect you to your own internal solutions; for we all hold the answers to our health and wellbeing, peace and happiness, within us; we heal from inside out. All remedies, no matter how potent or subtle, rely on the body's innate healing capacity and mechanisms; the most skilful surgeon or healer ultimately relies on the body's immune system and its intrinsic natural ability to repair, recover, and restore. Effective remedies may encourage and support this process. Also, when we proactively connect with and support each other we instigate an alchemic synergy; as previously acknowledged, like trees in a forest, we thrive and flourish when in positive communal connection with each other.

Healing and life support are multi-faceted processes. We resonate, our voice resonates (metabolic energy, the energy of intention, attitude, thoughts, meld into the vibration we emit). Plants resonate. When we talk to plants, it is not just the response of our voice and intention that influences the plant to potentially flourish, but also the carbon dioxide we emit from the breath we infuse into the plant's atmosphere, and in exchange, the respiring plant 'breathes' oxygen into ours.

We are designed to be well and to flourish; good health is the body's natural default state. We are sovereign beings gifted with life, just as nature (in its magnificence, beauty, and harshness) is sovereign too, inviting us to be consciously alive and aware, and sensually present in each moment, aiding our ability to thrive, providing nutrients, oxygen and medicine, and so much more, to enable us to recalibrate when we are 'out of sync'; colour, scents and visual beauty, and so much more.

Our body and nature work tirelessly to maintain a state of functional equilibrium; fostering and honouring this process makes perfect sense.

## 9. The rhythms and subtleties of nature

Nature and the environment around us are in constant flux and motion; the seasons, the weather, the atmosphere, the setting sun, the rising moon, and so on. We observe this movement and change as superficial, and internal, indicators with which we generally mark time (days, months, years, spring, summer, autumn, winter), manage growth and harvest, and so on. The ancients acknowledged this natural flux and flow as an expression of primordial energy; the omniscient quintessence of all organic and inorganic matter, living and non-living; vital energy, vital force, Prana (Hinduism), Ch'I (Qi) (Ancient Chinese), or élan vital (Western philosophy).

The literal translation of Ch'I, for example, is 'breath'; thus, we and everything materially manifest and unmanifest, are *breathed* into existence. Physically, breathing is a dualistic process: breath in, filling our lungs and, thus, every cell within our body, with vital life-sustaining oxygen; breath out, expelling carbon dioxide and spent metabolic debris. And so, the Ancient Chinese notion of yin (breath in) and yang (breath out) begins to formulate.

To elaborate this dynamic, yin and yang represent two polarised, opposing yet complementary forces, each perceivable by the contrasting existence of the other, lending shape, form and character to the material universe. While one dominates the other appears to yield, but dominance by either is never complete or constant – there always exists an element of yang in yin, and yin in yang (Godfrey 2019 p 171-173).

Similarly, Ayurveda (translated as 'life science' or 'knowledge of life'), the ancient Indian and Middle-Eastern life-style and healing (or recalibrating) system, also holds that creation issues from one all-pervading, omniscient, supreme spiritual energy, consciousness and intelligence (Prana), which manifests as three dynamical interplaying energetic qualities (generically referred to as 'doshas' - Vata, Pitta, and Kapha), that in motion give form to the material and ethereal; the mineral, plant and animal kingdom, atmosphere and the universe.  For example, Vata manifests as space and air and as the energy of activity, movement and mobility; Pitta manifests as fire and water and as the energy of transformation, digestion and metabolism; Kapha manifests as earth and water and as the energy of anabolism, growth and lubrication.

*See Ayurveda and the qualities of the three doshas Vatta, Pitta, and Kapha, and the Body Clock (Circadian Rhythm) and Elemental Characteristics charts in Appendix Two.*

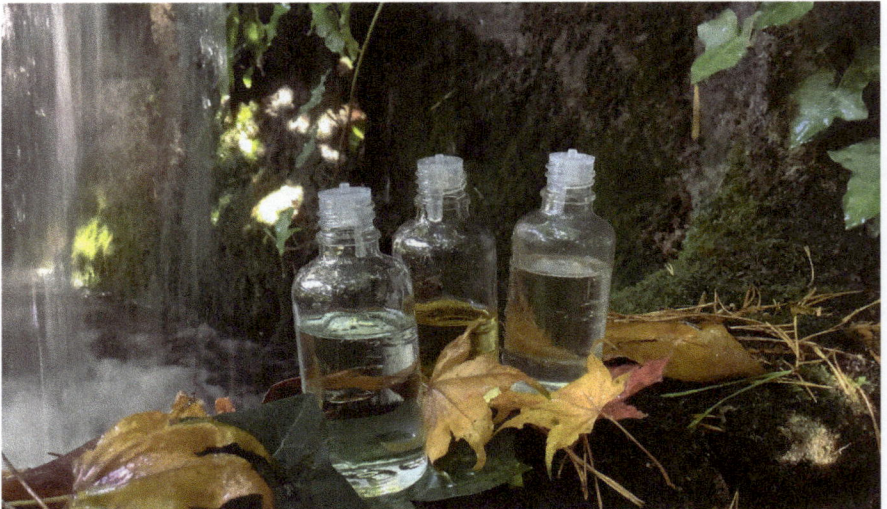

## 10. Observing seasonal change

Each season heralds atmospheric and environmental change in daylight, temperature and weather patterns, which in turn influence cycles of growth and harvest, activity and rest, and so on (for example, resting and dormant; stirring and new growth; blossoming and flowering; ripening, fruiting and harvesting). Our ancestors adhered to these cycles, eating seasonal foods, gathering available plant medicines, and seasonally relocating to optimal climatic environments. We are no longer nomadic, but we can tap into this innate rhythm to aid reunion with our own intrinsic connection with nature, to support our nourishment, equilibrium and recalibration as we traverse through each seasonal shift.

Seasons are cloaked in gradiating colours and shades. Light-dark cycles and seasons mark periods of change. Seasons are not strictly fixed to specific linear dates or periods; rather, they rhythmically 'pulse'. Our ancestors were acutely attuned to and responsive to the flux and flow, the rhythm and fluctuating motion of changing conditions and the seamless nuances of these nature-al 'pulses'. They instinctively related to, identified and responsively yielded to each season according to local hunting, gathering and climatic conditions, thus, aiding survival and flourishing.

While, today, we tend to refer to four relatively distinct calendar seasons (spring, summer, autumn and winter), our ancestors (depending on how close or far away from the equator they lived) acknowledged up to eight transient environmental states or periods. For example, Laplanders and Sami peoples (who inhabited the region of Sápmi, which encompassed northern areas now known as Finland, Norway, Russia, Sweden, Ukraine, Canada and the United States), acknowledge(d) four full and four half seasons: (1) autumn-winter; (2) winter; (3) spring-winter; (4) spring; (5) spring-summer; (6) summer; (7) summer-autumn; (8) autumn. Moon cycles were similarly identified; for example, moon of the long dark (late November early December), sun-wake moon (late December early January), willow grouse moon (late January early February), moon of the roaring rivers (late February early March), birchblood moon (late March early April), moon of the salmon run (late April early May), and so on (Paver 2020). Native American peoples observe(d) five seasons: (1) the budding of spring; (2) earing of corn or roasting time; (3) summer, or highest sun; (4) corn-gathering, or fall of the leaf; and, (5) winter, cry of wild geese (cohonk). They also acknowledge(d) thirteen moon cycles; for example, sugar moon or moon of the red grass appearing (April), flower moon or planting moon (May), blossom moon or green corn moon (June), and so on. *See the Native Indian Seasons and Moons chart in Appendix Two.*

Ancient Traditional Chinese Medicine (TCM) and Ayurveda, also the not-quite-so Ancient Greek and Roman physicians (for example, Hippocrates (c. 460 to 370 BC), Dioscorides (c. 40 to 90 AD), and Galen (c. 129 to 216 AD)), observe the flow of seasonal states and conditions and relate these with consequential seasonal disposition toward certain states of health and wellbeing. For example, according to Traditional Chinese Medicine, among other elemental qualities and conditions, winter is associated with water and yin energy, spring with wood and yang, summer with fire and yang, and autumn with metal and yin energy - the element earth grounds all seasons through transition from one state to another, thus the element earth possesses both yin and yang energy. Ayurveda associate autumn and winter with the characteristic quality of Kapha, spring with Vatta, and summer with Pitta.

Associated seasonal elements, bodily organ systems and conditions observed by our ancestors include:

**Winter:** cold and wet; fear, feeling scared, also positive feelings of calmness, patience, stability, happiness, compassion; the bladder and kidneys; the element water; the Chinese element Yin; the Galenic humour Phlegmatic; and the Ayurveda dosha Kapha.

**Spring:** cool and moist; anger, also positive feelings of creativity, enthusiasm and vitality; the liver and gall bladder; the element air (wind) or wood; the Chinese elements Yin and Yang; the humour Sanguine; and the Ayurveda dosha Vatta.

**Summer:** warm and dry; feeling happy, cheerful, courageous and contented; the heart and small intestine; the element fire; the Chinese element Yang; the Galenic humour Choleric; and the Ayurveda dosha Pitta.

**Autumn:** cool and dry; grief, feeling sad, also positive feelings of being grounded and earthed, calm and happy; the lungs and large intestines; the element earth or metal; the Chinese elements Yin and Yang; the Galenic humour Melancholic; and the Ayurveda dosha Kapha.

**Changing seasons** are associated with damp; feelings of love and compassion; the spleen and stomach; the element earth; the Chinese elements Yin and Yang; and the Ayurveda dosha Kapha.

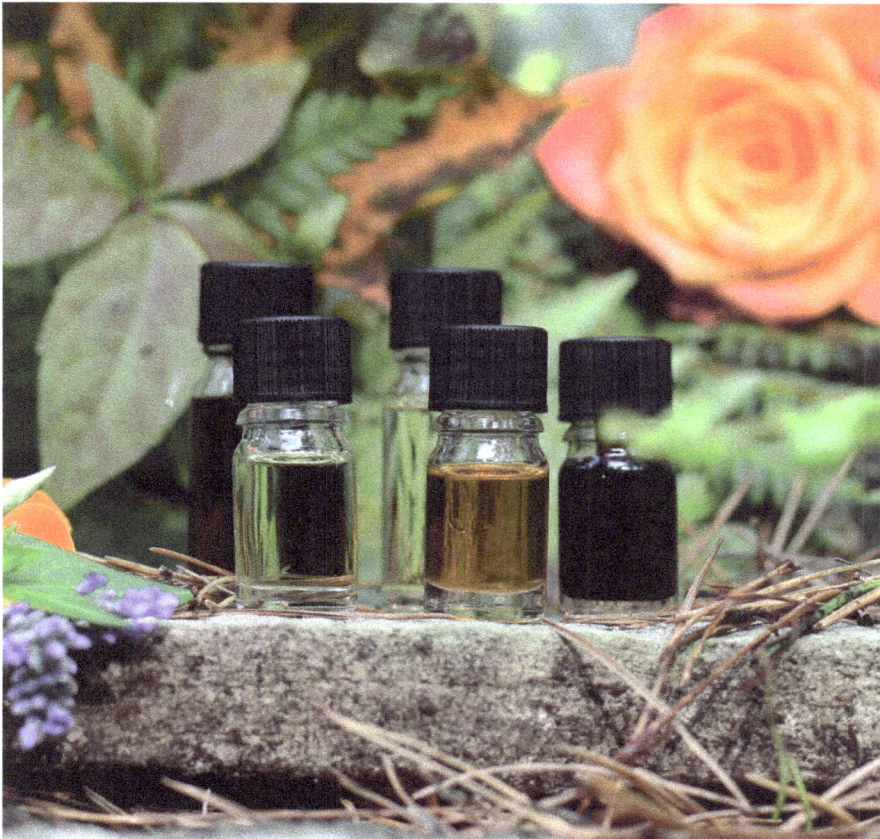

## 11. Seasonal affective or adjustment disorder (SAD)

Seasonal affective or adjustment disorder (SAD) is a type of depression, apparently more common in the West than the East, particularly in regions furthest from the Equator (Munir et al 2024; De Vaus et al 2017; Rosen et al 1990), and appears to be more prevalent in women than men, and highly sensitive individuals - HSP's. (Kuehner 2017; Chotia et al 2004; Farmer et al 2015). Symptoms may manifest during either late autumn / early winter, or late spring / early summer, usually in response to changing seasonal conditions (potentially triggered, for example, by diminishing or increased sunlight, ambient temperature reduction, and circadian rhythm disruption or changes, and so on). Indeed, according to traditional medicine, as observed above, autumn is associated with negative feelings or states of sadness (depression), winter with fear and feeling scared (anxiety) and spring with feelings of anger (inverted anger can express as depression and / or anxiety). Conversely, these seasons are also, as above and respectively, associated with positive productive states of mind and emotion, such as, intuition and rationality, resourcefulness and erudition, idealism and curiosity.

*See the Signs, Symptoms and Causes of Anxiety and Depression chart in Appendix One.*

## 12. Circadian Rhythms

There is increasing evidence linking circadian rhythmicity with change in mood, emotion, mental function and physical homeostasis. Disruption of circadian rhythms (whatever the cause) potentially upsets the body's metabolic equilibrium and regulatory processes.  In the short term, our body will adjust and recover balance.   However, when this disruption is continuous, the body can struggle to appropriately recalibrate; ongoing unaddressed disruption may pre-curse conditions such as seasonal adjustment disorder (as above), mood disorders, anxiety, depression, poor sleep patterns, poor digestion and poor assimilation of vital nutrients, and weakened immune system function.

Natural light plays a significant role in regulation and balance of the body's 'clock' mechanism.  Clock genes are found inside cells throughout the body and, through activation of various positive and negative feedback loops, identify the time of day according to the amount of available light. Clock genes set a series of related responses into motion; for example, sleep-wake cycles and metabolic synchronicity involving hormone release, cardiovascular and renal function, digestion, hepatic-metabolism and so on. A vital component of the body's self-healing and regulatory mechanisms, sleep allows the body to build up stored energy, to remodel neurones for synaptic function, to facilitate newly acquired memory consolidation and assimilation, which includes memory consolidation of complex motor systems that facilitate coordination, motion and movement of the body (spinal cord, brain stem, primary motor cortex and nervous system), and facilitation of tissue healing, repair and restoration, among other things.

There are four circadian clock cycles:

• **Diurnal:** Daytime and night-time activity; for example, regulation of daytime and night-time temperature.

• **Circadian:** Twenty-four-hour; for example, pineal gland stimulation (melatonin), and secretion of cortisol and insulin.

• **Ultradian:** Less than twenty-four-hours; for example, energetic optimisation and internal co-ordination, such as, alternating periods of high-frequency brain activity (about ninety minutes) followed by lower-frequency brain activity (about twenty minutes); we notice this when we suddenly cannot concentrate or focus, need to switch from cerebral tasks to physical activity, or to rest – make a cup of tea, be still for a moment.

• **Infradian/Circaluna** (one month/seasonal); for example, regulation of mood, reproduction and growth cycles, adjusting to seasonal changes, stress responses, immune system efficiency and microbiome activity.

Being aware of the flux of the body's regulatory mechanisms, of seasonal transience and associated environmental conditions and the potential consequential physiological and psycho-emotional-spiritual influence these rhythms invite, affords us foresight that allows us to prepare and compensate, and to operate in positive synchronicity.

*See the Body Clock (Circadian Rhythm) and Elemental Characteristics and the Chinese Medicine Body Clock, Elements and Essential Oils charts in Appendix Two.*

## 13. Meditation and the locus of conscious control

Meditation, like prayer, visualisation, chanting and dance, is an ancient practice.

Meditation returns and gently sustains conscious awareness to the moment, so we are centred within the present. Indeed, everything we need and can handle in life is present-ed to us one moment at a time. Meditation enables you to stand (or consciously 'be') at the centre of each moment and observe, and thus, gain a greater sense of awareness of what is, and to master the conscious ability to 'respond' rather than 'react'. Breath focus, a technique of meditation, is a simple practice which features as an aspect of many disciplines, ancient and modern, from yoga and prayer, to the practice of relaxation techniques.

The outcome of meditation is often very subtle. Initially, there is a sense of calm, then, as we get on with our daily lives, we may notice that we naturally respond, rather than react, to thoughts and events with a gentle sense of control. Our attitude may alter; for example, the glass may become half-full instead of half-empty. We may become more aware and aligned with our bodily sensations, and more readily notice the nuances of change and motion in the rhythm and flow. We may actively listen, and consciously speak. When we are disturbed, for whatever reason, we are better able to move through the experience and return to a sense of equilibrium. We may also feel a sense of contentment for no reason other than that we are simply content. Past regrets, traumas or disappointments, even memory of joy and pleasure, future fears, uncertainty, anxiety, anticipation, and expectations, are disarmed, disempowered, when we consciously stand at the epicentre of 'present moment' awareness.

However, although incredibly simple, meditation (staying consciously 'in the moment') can sometimes appear to be the hardest thing to do. For example, I can find time, create space, and sit with every good intention to formally meditate... then, suddenly, I wonder if I turned the oven off, I become aware of the clock ticking in the next room, my mind drifts along the threads of whispered thoughts and musings. Do not despair! This is what the mind does, and continues to do, even when we are asleep. Notice its rambling, but do not give it your attention. Instead, focus your awareness on your breath as it rises and falls within, and allow your minds incessant chatter to drift to the side-line: observe, notice, acknowledge, but remain consciously aware of your breathing; thus, we sit 'within', patiently, compassionately, at the gateway, aware of 'being'.

Equally, meditation is not a magic wand that waves all our cares away and whisks up our 'happily ever after'. It may still rain on your wedding day; your flight may still be cancelled as you are about to embark on the holiday of a lifetime; you may not win the game, or get the promotion you hoped for.   Meditation, however, is initially a little bit like 'rewilding the soul'; an over-ploughed and depleted field, abandoned and barren of life after years of repeatedly growing the same crop, left to its own devices will suddenly begin to bloom again as nature magnificently reclaims its territory. In rediscovering our own magnificence, we then notice that life is full of miracles that completely outshine rain on our wedding day.

You will find deeper detail about the practice, process and nuances of meditation in my book, *Essential Oils for Mindfulness and Meditation (2019)*.

Visualisation is another useful tool. Through conscious visualisation we are able to deliberately and sensually conjure pleasant images; to positively redress and reframe memories and past experiences, or present worries and anxieties; to colour or re-colour the picture of our inner reflection, our imagining, to assemble the pieces and fragments in a different light, to positively recalibrate negative thoughts and feelings.  Returning our focus, our awareness, to the moment, we are bathed in the sensual experience ignited by this facet of our imagination; the threads of our past tapestry, concerns or negative feelings, no longer pulling at the threads of the present masterful creation.

Writing in a personal journal is another potential tool. This can be done in a structured themed way (what made me smile today? and so on) or as unconditional free-flow: a clean page, pen in hand, pen to paper as thoughts, feelings, images emerge.  Free-flow writing is a useful way to reveal and reflect on subconscious insights and messages, and can also be cathartic; that is, in musing, in allowing my inner self to freely pour onto the page, I release the stopper from the bottle, my thoughts and feelings are able to flow from me instead of perpetually rattling around inside me like a pea in a drum in ever exaggerated loudness or colour. The process of free-flow writing is like creating a hologram that I can see through from different angles and perspectives.  My reflection and observation allow me to incline toward being 'master' rather than 'servant'.

Setting goals is a useful strategy to recapture a sense of control. However, I have observed that during times of very high anxiety making to-do lists can intensify a sense of overwhelm or burden rather than soothe and placate; meditation, visualisation or writing in a journal may have a similar effect for the same reason.  Indeed, I have noticed that at these times, any attention or focus on my mental chatter, or my inner feelings and sensations, even my breath, appears to magnify and increase my anxiety. During these moments, physical activity and focus on practical tasks enables me to channel my excessive anxious mental energy: this is not an act of surrendering to avoidance; in carefully choosing my moments I take control, I remain 'master' not 'servant'.  Reaching for my essential oils is, thankfully, another supportive strategy during such times.

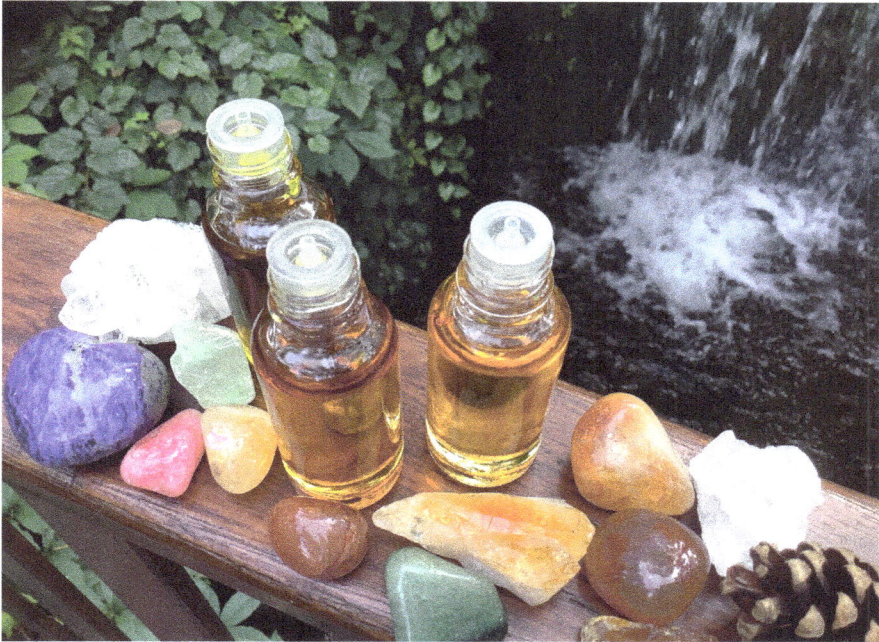

## 14. Essential oils to ease anxiety
## - reviewing the science

E ssential oils are, indeed, gifts of nature.

Sensually observing the scent of essential oils, or the plants they are present within, we are aware of our breathing, we willingly linger in the moment. Applied to support meditation, essential oils may aid focus and concentration, wakefulness, instil a sense of peace and calm, uplift mood and emotion, aid memory, inspire a sense of grounded pleasure and joy, or simply clear the sinuses and ease breathing.

Indeed, essential oils possess multiple supportive qualities that instigate various responses within the body, the most significant in terms of meditation (prayer or visualisation) and in terms of quelling anxiety, is their direct influence on the organs of the limbic system (the instinctive and emotional centre within the brain, which incorporates the amygdala, hippocampus, thalamus and hypothalamus), and their indirect influence on the pituitary gland (thus, consequently, endocrine hormones), and the frontal lobe (simply, the area of the brain that helps us 'make sense' of things) Essential oil molecules interact with olfactory receptors found, not only in the nasal cavities, but also in other tissues and organs throughout the body. These neural signals are activated when essential oil molecules are absorbed into the body's circulatory system a) via alveoli in the lungs, respiratory tract, and soft tissue in the roof of the nasal cavity, b) via dermal application, and c) via consumption of foods.

Essential oils diffused during meditation (prayer, visualization or relaxation) can also be employed (perhaps applied in a perfume or cream or environmental incense) to act as a reminder, to bring forward, to re-instil within the moment, the memory of the experience felt during formal meditation (there and then) 'here and now', thus effectively compounding positive feelings and encouraging us to perpetuate moment-centred consciousness.

(Godfrey 2022, 2019 and 2018)

Sowndhararajan et al (2016), for example, carried out a comprehensive systematic review of published literature to evaluate the influence of plant-derived and synthetic fragrance on human psychophysiological activity. Direct inhalation of fragrances, they conclude, even a small amount, demonstrates significant effect on brain activity. This, they concur, is due to the ability of odour compounds to cross the blood-brain barrier and interact with receptors within the limbic system, pituitary gland, frontal lobe and wider central nervous system. Inhalation of scent molecules produced immediate changes in physiological parameters, such as blood pressure, muscle tension, pupil dilation, skin temperature, pulse rate and skin activity, memory and recall. Essential oils and other fragrant compounds cited by Sowndhararajan et al, that demonstrate cephalic and central nervous system influence, include, among others, bergamot, caraway, chamomile, eucalyptus, geranium, grapefruit, jasmine, lemongrass, lavender, neroli, palmarosa, peppermint, pine and rosemary. For example, rose, jasmine and lavender were shown to attenuate blood pressure; lavender reduced mental stress and improved deep sleep; rose and patchouli caused significant decrease (up to forty per cent) in sympathetic nervous system activity; rosemary improved overall quality of memory; peppermint reduced fatigue, improved mood and decreased daytime sleepiness; orange and lavender reduced anxiety; lavender, chamomile, rosemary and lemon, combined with massage, reduced anxiety and improved self-esteem; chamomile Roman demonstrated sedative effects.

Soto-Vasquez et al (2016), in a study exploring the effect of mindfulness meditation and the psycho-emotional influence of essential oils, found that, when combined, essential oils and meditation appear to act synergistically (one enhancing or potentiating the effect of the other), and significantly reduce levels of anxiety. The essential oils applied in this study (Satureja brevicalyx and Satureja boliviana – plants native to Peru) contain a high content of linalool, a phyto-chemical attributed with being 'uplifting', among other qualities, which, the authors suggest, contributed to the outcome. They also acknowledge that other essential oils containing linalool may potentially produce a similar effect and suggest a blend of Ho wood, geranium and peppermint (peppermint oil does not contain linalool, but in combination these oils create a similar chemical 'fingerprint' to the Peruvian oils). Basil (linalool CT), lavender, neroli and petitgrain also contain high levels of linalool.

In another literature review, which explored linalool as a therapeutic and medicinal tool applied in the treatment of depression, Santos et al (2022) similarly observe the positive supportive bioactive influence of this compound on several neurological pathways related to depression. Linalool's influence on the monoaminergic system, which involves neurotransmitters such as serotonin, dopamine, norepinephrine, epinephrine and histamine, indicates several possible mechanisms by which linalool expresses an anti-depressant effect, justifying its significance as a promising integrative tool in the treatment of depression. Lavender *angustifolia* essential oil contains a high percentage of both linalool (up to forty-five per cent) and linalyl acetate (up to forty-five per cent). Other essential oils mentioned in this review, either due to their high linalool content, or their blending compatibility with lavender and/or linalool, include: bergamot, coriander, caraway, clary sage, neroli, rosemary, and ylang ylang.

Poignantly, Tan et al (2023) in their study, which involved analysis of forty-four randomised controlled trials, found that essential oil therapy led to a significant reduction of both state and trait anxiety, with a more obvious effect on state anxiety and a stabilising effect on trait anxiety. Of the ten essential oils that formed the focus of this study, jasmine (*Jasminum sambac* (L.), which contains a moderate amount of *linalool*, among many other compatible constituents, was the essential oil most recommended for treating state anxiety, followed closely by bitter orange (*citrus aurantium* L.), which contains high amounts of d-limonene and low amounts of *linalool*, then rose Damask (*Rosa x damascene*), which contains moderately high amounts of *citronellol, nerol* and *geraniol*, and small amounts of *linalool*, among many other compatible constituents, and mint (*mentha piperita*), which contains moderately high amounts of *menthone* and *menthol*; mint stimulates the hypothalamus to instigate a parasympathetic response, which in turn reduces anxiety. Lavender (*Lavandula angustifolia*), which contains high amounts of *linalool* and *linalyl acetate* (as acknowledged previously), demonstrated efficacy for both state and trait anxiety. Other essential oils included lemon (*Citrus limon*) and geranium (*Palargonium graveolenes*), bushy matgrass (*Lippia alba Mill*) and Lemon Verbena (*Lippia citriodora*), and copaiba (*Copaifera officinalis*).

Although lemon, geranium, bushy matgrass and lemon verbena essential oils did not demonstrate high anti-anxiety efficacy in this study, other studies do support their anxiolytic benefits (Seo et al 2023, Ozer et al 2022, Alvardo-Garcia et al 2021, Sherzadegan et al 2017). Copaiba demonstrated no anxiolytic benefits in this study, however, again, other studies do support this oil's anti-anxiety effects (Zhang et al 2022).

- Serotonin acts as a hormone that carries messages between nerve cells within the brain (the central nervous system) and throughout the body (the peripheral nervous system).

- Histamine is a chemical of the immune system, which among other roles, regulates the sleep-wake cycle and cognitive function.

- Dopamine influences areas of the brain involved with feelings of satisfaction, motivation and pleasure, and also plays a part in controlling memory, mood, sleep, learning, concentration, movement and other body functions.

- Noradrenaline plays an essential role in regulation of arousal, attention, cognitive function, and stress reactions.

- Adrenaline is a hormone and a neurotransmitter that plays an important role in the 'flight or fright' response and feelings of fear and anxiety.

- Cortisol is the primary stress hormone and slows functions that would be nonessential or harmful in a fight or flight situation. Cortisol increases sugar (glucose) in the blood stream, enhances the brain's use of glucose and increases the availability of substances in the body that repair tissues.

I do not advocate the internal use of essential oils. However, there is evidence that herbal teas, which contain essential oils, among other compounds (such as, alkaloids, bitters and flavonoids) and trace elements, may be beneficial. For example, Roman chamomile tea is shown to aid sleep and reduce anxiety (Jia et al 2021, Srivastava 2010); rosemary tea eases anxiety and depression (Achour et al 2022, Ferlemi et al 2015), similarly, so do lavender tea (Bazrafshan et al 2020), and lemon balm (melissa) tea (Ghazizadeh et al 2021); whilst peppermint tea eases stress and insomnia (Caro et al 2018). Peppermint and chamomile tea also ease digestive problems (dyspepsia); an 'upset tummy' is another co-morbidity associated with anxiety (Vasey 2006).

Essential oils are adaptogens (that is, they support the body's response to stress, anxiety and fatigue, and encourage feelings of wellbeing) and tend to normalise or balance rather than simply stimulate or sedate. They instigate physiological, endocrine, neural and psycho-emotional responses. They are physiologically and psycho-emotionally protective, restorative, rejuvenating, calming and sedating, uplifting and stimulating. In terms of the influence of essential oils on anxiety, agitation and restlessness, for example, the scent of cedarwood Atlas instils feelings of peace; frankincense and patchouli slow and deepen breathing, instilling a sense of ease and calmness; myrrh revitalises and stimulates, yet at the same time is also calming; spikenard protects the heart (pericardium) and instils a sense of tranquillity. Significantly, these, among other essential oils, are also anti-inflammatory (for example, carrot seed, chamomile, helichrysum, frankincense, geranium, lavender, melissa, myrrh, lemongrass, patchouli, peppermint, sandalwood, spikenard and turmeric).

Chronic anxiety is linked with systemic inflammation which is apparently shown in turn to pre-curse autoimmune, lung and cardiovascular diseases and gastrointestinal disorders; for example, arthritis, asthma, high blood pressure, heart disease and inflammatory bowel disease (and vice versa, these conditions may instigate feelings of anxiety) (Sattayakhom et al 2023, Kennedy and Niedzwidz 2022, Ravi et al 2021, Michopoulas et al 2017, Vogelzangs et al 2013).

Essential oils may also:

**Aid focus and concentration** – for example, cajeput, carrot seed, cypress, hyssop, lemon, lemongrass, niaouli, orang bitter, peppermint, petitgrain, rosemary, tea tree and thyme.

**Aid wakefulness** – for example, cajeput, ginger, lemongrass, pepper black, peppermint, rosemary and tea tree.

**Aid sleep** *(in small amounts)* – for example, sweet basil, bergamot, chamomile Roman, coriander, frankincense, geranium, juniper, lavender, marjoram, mandarin, may chang, melissa, myrtle, neroli, orange bitter, petitgrain, rose, spikenard, thyme, valerian, vetivert, yarrow and ylang ylang.

**Reduce feelings of addiction** – for example, grapefruit and vetivert.

**Aid a sense of balance and control** – for example, cedarwood Atlas, bergamot, chamomile Roman, cypress, frankincense, galbanum, geranium, juniper berry, lavender, lemon, mandarin, marjoram, orange bitter, patchouli, and spikenard.

**Aid a sense of self-confidence** – for example, cajeput, jasmine, lemongrass, neroli (orange blossom), sweet marjoram, melissa (lemon balm), rose Otto, sage clary and rosemary.

**Aid a sense of feeling grounded** – for example, cedarwood, fennel, myrrh, patchouli, black pepper, spikenard, thyme linalool, turmeric and vetivert.

**Calm agitation** – for example, bergamot, carrot seed, cedarwood Atlas, chamomile Roman, frankincense, lavender, jasmine, melissa (lemon balm), orange bitter, palmarosa, patchouli, rose otto, sandalwood, spikenard, valerian and vetivert.

**Uplift mood** – for example, basil, bergamot, cardamom, citronella, clove bud, galbanum, geranium, grapefruit, jasmine, juniper berry, lavender, lemon, mandarin, may chang, orange bitter, neroli (orange blossom), peppermint, petitgrain, rose Otto, rosemary, thyme, yarrow and ylang ylang.

Clearly, essential oils make for wonderful 'travelling' companions.

*See The psycho-emotional qualities of sixty essential oils below.*

## 15. Essential oils and the seasons: aligning their potential

Seasonal patterns vary across the world.

For example, December, January and February incorporate winter season in Britain but summer in Australia. Observing British seasonal months as an anchor point, the following are examples of essential oils harvested and extracted during:

**Winter:** Citrus fruits, cedarwood, myrrh, turmeric and ylang ylang.

**Spring:** Geranium, neroli, black pepper, rose, spikenard, tea tree, thyme and valerian.

**Summer:** Carrot seed, chamomiles, hyssop, jasmine, melissa, myrrh, peppermint, petitgrain, pine needle, nutmeg, rosemary, clary sage, and yarrow.

**Autumn:** Cardamon, coriander, fennel, grapefruit, juniper berry, neroli, marjoram, may chang, spikenard, turmeric and valerian.

Some plants are harvested and distilled during both spring and autumn, for example, neroli blossoms and myrrh, and some are harvested all year-round, especially trees, such as sandalwood, frankincense, clove and cinnamon, and plants and fruits, such as, lemongrass and lemons.

Cypress is harvested and distilled during autumn, winter and early spring. Cypress essential oil aids transition through these seasons and encourages us to walk tall into spring as we move out of winters cave; cypress supports change, 'moving on' and 'letting go', and eases feelings of anxiety, fear and grief, and feelings of being 'stuck'.

Essential oils that bring sunshine and warmth to short bleak winter days include uplifting and vitalising citrus oils, such as, bergamot, grapefruit, lemon, mandarin and orange, and warming drying oils, such as cedarwood, myrrh, black pepper, turmeric and ylang ylang.  Lemon-scented essential oils, such as, melissa (lemon balm) and lemongrass, may also ease winter blues. Also, spice oils, such as, cinnamon, clove and nutmeg are strong anti-microbial essential oils and added to orange or grapefruit oil create wonderful anti-microbial room scents that add spice and warmth to cold days. Frankincense and myrrh have 'earthing', warming, drying, antimicrobial and calming qualities; they support the immune system, stave off colds and 'flu, and act as antidotes to the dampness of winter; combined with bitter orange or another citrusy oil, they can at the same time dispel feelings of anxiety and depression.  Mandarin and the earthy-smoky scent of vetivert, combined with the sweet rose-like scent of geranium express similar uplifting yet grounding qualities, and may also aid in alleviating conditions such as anxiety, depression and seasonal adjustment disorder (SAD).

Essential oils that aid, or support, transition from one season to another (or one situation or condition to another) include:

**From spring to summer:** Cypress, rose and lavender.

**From summer to autumn:** Melissa (lemon balm), petitgrain, pine needle and nutmeg.

**From autumn to winter:** Coriander, juniper berry, marjoram and turmeric.

**From winter to spring:** Cedarwood, citrus fruit oils, myrrh, black pepper, vetivert and ylang ylang.

Also, grouping types of essential oils together as a very general guide, or starting point, may aid selection when applying generic qualities of essential oils. For example:

Woods and flowers or blossoms in combination tend to be balancing and uplifting.

Woods tend to aid breathing.

Resins and roots tend to be grounding or 'earthing'.

Spices and citrus oils tend to be stimulating, wakening and brightening.

Herbs tend to be balancing; some are more stimulating than others (rosemary, for example), some more relaxing (marjoram, for example), some are both stimulating and relaxing (lavender and patchouli, for example).

*See the Seasons, Direction and Ancient Wisdom chart, and the Chinese Medicine Body Clock, Elements, and Essential Oils chart, also the Essential Oil-Bearing Plants and Optimal Harvest Times and Related Seasons chart in Appendix Two.*

The sense of smell is idiosyncratic and, thus, very personal. What one person likes, another may respond to indifferently or dislike. Even rose, famously the most beautiful floral oil, is repugnant to some people – too sweet, too sickly. You cannot be certain, when you proudly adorn your beautiful perfume creation, that others around you will be as enthusiastic as you are about the scent. Also, remember, we exude our own bodily scent which, when mingled with perfumes or essential oils, can render a scent as something quite different from the perfume in the bottle; the whisp of perfume that you may have noticed on the person passing you by, or standing next to you in a lift, may consequently elude you when trying to source or replicate it. This also applies when we create ambient room scents; other people in the room will observe differing qualities, tones and notes, according to their needs and perception, their state of health, their age, their memories and the efficiency of their olfactory receptors.

The beauty of an essential oil is that as the molecules that formulate it, or the blend of oils, begin to drift from the mixture, its 'tune' gently changes until it naturally fades, just as nature intended; unlike synthetic scents, which remain fixed and almost static. The scent of an essential oil is dynamic, the complex mixture of various odour 'notes' are mobile; the symphony you begin with dwindles to a gently lingering sinfonia as time drifts by.

When applying essential oils, it is advisable to start with a single essential oil or a simple themed blend, and to gradually build your repertoire as you become experientially familiar with their multiple exuding qualities and characteristics.  For example, when creating an environmental ambience, perhaps to bring a whisp of nature into the square room in the square building you inhabit, scents can be selectively chosen to instigate a particular sensual impression or image.  Maybe, for example, meandering through an English garden (lavender, chamomile, melissa, clary sage, yarrow, peppermint); a Mediterranean citrus grove (petitgrain, neroli, orange, lemon, cypress, thyme, marjoram, helichrysum); a summer-drenched woodland (cedarwood, birch, galbanum, carrot seed, rosemary); a northern forest (pine and juniper); a middle eastern valley (frankincense, myrrh, rose, geranium, mint); an Indian market (sandalwood, patchouli, turmeric, cinnamon, cardamon, lemongrass, spikenard); an oriental courtyard (jasmine, ylang ylang, may Chang), and so on.  Essential oils are pleasantly hedonistic, uplifting, grounding, soothing, relaxing, inspiring, stimulating, awakening, brightening, and gently, sensually, stir mood, emotion and imagination; they are also anti-microbial and thus protective and healing.

*See the Scent Groups, and Essential Oil Scent Profile charts in Appendix Two.*

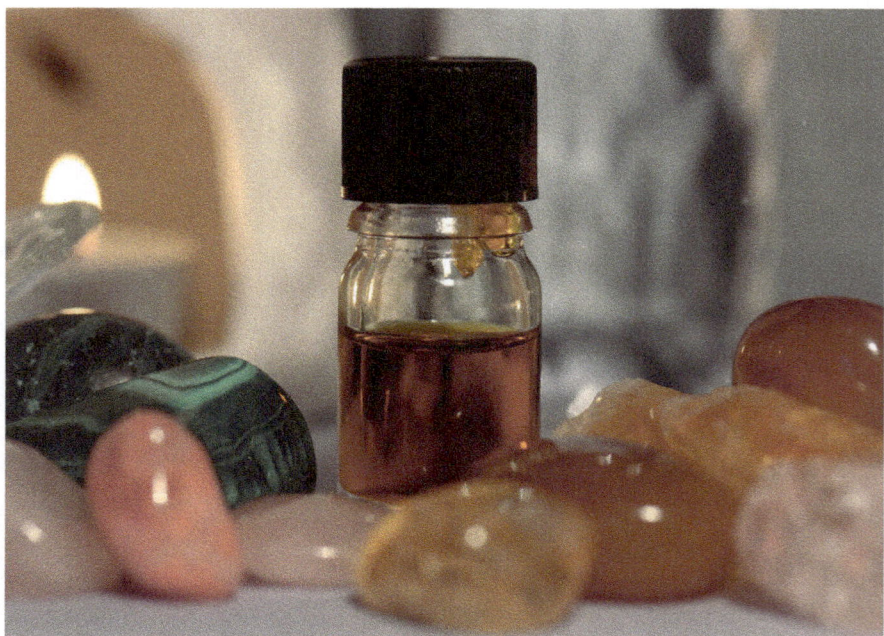

# Applying Essential Oils

*Now we come to the practical part.*

*In this section we take a further brief look at what essential oils are to better comprehend their nature and how to apply them safely and effectively. Essential oils that potentially ease feelings of anxiety are then identified, followed by an overview of the psycho-emotional qualities of sixty commonly used essential oils, and then safe measurement guidelines and instruction about methods of application. Using the preceding insight about the various dynamics, properties and qualities of essential oils, along with the information below and the information in the appendix, you can hone your choice to suit your specific personal requirement with precision.*

## 16. What are essential oils?  A brief overview

Essential oils comprise a highly concentrated mixture of various volatile organic chemical compounds (mainly terpenes and their terpenoid derivatives) that are extracted from trees and plants, such as the whole plant of geranium or bitter fennel, or parts of plants, such as leaves, fruits, flowers, bark, resin, sawdust, roots and so on.

While essential oils demonstrate some of the qualities exhibited by the plant, the process of extracting and removing the essential oil from the plant alters its chemical composition and scent profile. For example, many of the oils non-distillable, non-volatile and hydrophilic (water-loving) components are either left behind in the plant material, or bond with water molecules and/or oxygen molecules within the atmosphere during the process of extraction, or separation, from the plant material (steam or water distillation, or in the case of fruit rinds, expression – crushing).

Also, the heat and pressure applied during steam distillation influence the chemical presentation of the resultant essential oil; some molecules transform during this process, sometimes creating components that are not present within the plant. Matricin, one example, a colourless sesquiterpene molecule found in chamomile, wormwood and yarrow, is biosynthesised during distillation to form the blue-violet compound chamazulene, which does not exist in the plant.

Thus, essential oils, when removed from the plant, are ultimately rendered the unique product of extraction. They are highly concentrated isolates (fifty to a hundred times more concentrated in a bottle than when present in a single plant). For example, it takes thirty-five pounds of lavender flowers to produce just fifteen millilitres of essential oil (or approximately three hundred drops), and two thousand five hundred to four thousand kilograms of rose petals to produce just one kilogram of rose essence. Just one drop of essential oil is equivalent to fifteen to forty cups of medicinal tea or up to ten teaspoons of tincture.

Essential oils mainly comprise of hydrophobic / lipophilic (water-hating / fat-loving) compounds. While some water compatible components bond with oxygen molecules within water, essential oils generally do not dissolve or disperse in water; their molecules will cluster together and float on the surface of water, or will sink if denser and heavier than water (for example, vetiver and myrrh tend to sink when dropped into water). While they are oil-like in their behaviour (that is, they do not mix with water), essential oils are not 'greasy' or 'oily', like fat or vegetable oils (which are also known as 'fixed oil's'); therefore, they are not lubricant and are, in fact, extremely drying and potentially irritating to the skin, even in small quantities. This is why drops of essential oils are always blended in an emollient substance, such as a vegetable oil, ointment, cream or lotion, when applied to the body.

Emollients can also add their own unique skin supporting qualities when considerately blended with essential oils to create very effective skincare synergies.

Essential oil molecules more readily leave, or partition, from a water-based medium (for example, lotions, creams and gels) to bond with lipids in the skin, rather than from an oily medium or ointment. However, vegetable oils and ointments create a barrier that prevents or significantly decreases water evaporation from skin, which increases opportunity for essential oil molecules to penetrate; essential oil molecules must be in direct contact with skin to be absorbed.

When prescribed by a herbalist or doctor for internal ingestion, essential oils are applied in small controlled amounts, contained in a dispersant emollient and/or within a 'safe to swallow' gel-like – preferably vegetable – capsule (composed of hypromellose, a polymer formulated from plant cellulose); the animal version (gelatine) is derived from skin or bone collagen (not suitable for vegans or vegetarians). Essential oils are not recommended for internal ingestion unless prescribed and/or administered by a professional healthcare practitioner or herbalist who has appropriate knowledge of the chemical constituents of essential oils and how these interact with bodily enzymes and chemicals, and other prescribed chemicals found in medications that may be being taken at the same time.

Employing their antimicrobial, skin and underlying soft tissue healing qualities, essential oils may be safely** and effectively applied topically to skin in appropriate dilution in vegetable oil* or vegetable wax* (for example, jojoba), gels (such as aloe vera gel, or gels made from pectin or cellulose gum, among others, and distilled water), ointment* and compresses, to treat local conditions, such as eczema, sprains, insect bites, to aid repair of damaged skin tissue, improve the appearance of scars, and to combat minor infections. Essential oils are also added to creams and lotions for their cleansing, toning and other skincare qualities. Essential oils may also be applied topically (as a compress, or essential oil-infused cream, lotion or vegetable oil) to mid or lower back and/or abdomen, to aid the digestive system and reproductive organs; for example, to alleviate indigestion, symptoms of IBS, or to ease menstrual pain, and so on.

Essential oils are also effectively applied, in dilution and small quantity (one to four drops of essential oil), via inhalation using, for example, drops on a tissue or cotton pad, aroma sticks (specially designed nasal inhalers), 'therapeutic perfumes' (for example, diluted in vegetable oil and dispensed using a roller bottle), and steam inhalation, or a room diffuser; respectively applied to relieve the symptoms of a cold or sore throat, or for their psycho-emotional benefits (uplifting, calming, energising), or as an ambient room scent, and so on.

*The antiseptic action of phenols (components found in clove, cinnamon, basil, and thyme, for example – note that phenol rich essential oils tend to be skin irritants) are possibly negated by fatty or oily mediums (Bensouilah and Buck 2006 p 75 - 76).

**Always check the qualities and safety information of an essential oil before applying it.

Ensure your essential oils are derived from a sustainable source; especially, for example, spikenard and frankincense, also rosewood and sandalwood; if you cannot find a sustainable source, you may, for example, substitute spikenard with vetivert or valerian, and frankincense with patchouli or myrrh.

## 17. Essential oils, our sense of smell, and the limbic system

When we sniff or smell an essential oil, its scent molecules (terpenes and terpenoids) are detected (like a key in a lock) by olfactory receptors located at the top of each nasal cavity that, in turn, relay nerve impulses to the Limbic System located in the brain. Odour receptors are also located in other areas of the body, such as the skin and other organs (heart, liver, lungs, kidneys and gastrointestinal tract).  However, by grand design, it seems, proximity of the master olfactory portal in the roof of the nasal cavity ensures immediate awareness and instinctive reflexive responses.

The Limbic System incorporates various functional structures located in the central paleomammalian area of the brain (which include the amygdala, hippocampus and hypothalamus) that are responsible for basic physiological and emotional responses to sensory stimulation. The hypothalamus functionally connects the Limbic System to the frontal lobe (where the brain rationalises and makes sense of information and sensory input) and to the pituitary gland. The pituitary gland, also known as the master endocrine gland, initiates hormone release in response to sensory signals, activating either the sympathetic or parasympathetic nervous system, depending on the nature of the stimuli.  As discussed earlier, the sympathetic nervous system prepares the body for 'fight or flight' (protection), and the parasympathetic nervous system maintains a state of peace and relaxation (rest and digest), and disengages the sympathetic nervous system post 'alert', returning the body to its optimal functional resting state.

When inhaled, in addition to affecting the olfactory sense, some essential oil molecules may also be transported via the bloodstream, to the brain by crossing the blood brain barrier. Here they may interact with various receptor sites, such as, GABA (gamma-aminobutyric acid) and glutamate receptors, located in the hippocampus, thalamus, basal ganglia, hypothalamus, and brainstem (GABA is an amino acid that functions to reduce neuronal excitability by inhibiting nerve transmission).  (Cui et al 2022, Soares et al 2022, Fung et al 2021, Wu et al 2009)

The mechanisms by which essential molecules are absorbed and interact within the body are very complex and, although modern technology affords much insight, are still not fully realised.  However, our body is clearly 'wired' to receive phyto-molecules; as verified by the presence of numerous (olfactory and endocannabinoid) receptor sites scattered throughout the body and the multilateral physical and psychosomatic responses instigated by detection.

(Godfrey 2022, 2020, 2019)

For deeper insight about the composition, properties and qualities of essential oils please refer to *Healing with Essential Oils and Essential Oils for the Whole Body.*

The following charts list various emotional states linked with the experience of anxiety, and depression, and essential oils that may help alleviate these states.

## 18. Essential oils to ease anxiety and balance mood and emotion

*A quick 'at a glance' guide*

| Grounding | Calming / Balancing | Uplifting |
|---|---|---|
| **Benzoin, cardamom, carrot seed, cedarwood, chamomile(s),** clove bud, **coriander, frankincense, helichrysum, jasmine, myrrh, neroli,** nutmeg, **palmarosa, patchouli,** petitgrain, **rose otto, rose absolute, sandalwood, spikenard,** thyme (red), **turmeric, valerian, vetivert, ylang ylang** | **Angelica root, bergamot,** cajeput, caraway, **cardamom, carrot seed, chamomile(s), chaste tree,** cinnamon, **cypress, fennel, frankincense, galbanum, geranium, ginger, grapefruit, helichrysum,** hyssop, **jasmine, juniper berry, lavender(s),** lemongrass, **marjoram, melissa (lemon balm),** myrtle, **neroli, palmarosa, patchouli,** black pepper, **peppermint, petitgrain,** pine, **rose otto,** rosemary, **clary sage,** thyme (white), **sandalwood, spikenard,** yarrow | **Basil, bergamot,** cajeput, clove bud, citronella, eucalyptus, **frankincense, galbanum, grapefruit,** lavender spike, **lemon, mandarin, may chang, melissa (lemon balm),** niaouli, nutmeg, **bitter orange,** oregano, **palmarosa, peppermint, petitgrain,** pine, **rose otto,** rosemary, **clary sage,** tea tree, **turmeric,** yarrow, turpentine, **ylang ylang** |

## 19. Anxiety and it's wider scope - complementary essential oils

*A quick 'at a glance' guide*

| Condition | Signature essential oils to ease | Supporting essential oils |
|---|---|---|
| **Agitation / Restlessness** | Basil (French, Sweet), cedarwood Atlas, chamomile Roman and German, frankincense, lavender, mandarin, marjoram, neroli (orange blossom), bitter orange, palmarosa, patchouli, petitgrain, sandalwood, spikenard, valerian, vetivert. | Carrot seed, helichrysum, juniper berry, melissa (lemon balm), myrrh, yarrow. |
| **Addiction** (see also *Moving on*) | Grapefruit, juniper berry, vetivert | Frankincense, carrot seed, cypress |
| **Anger** | Bergamot, cedarwood Atlas, chamomile(s), cypress, frankincense, geranium, lavender, myrtle, petitgrain, rose | Spikenard, yarrow |
| **Apathy** (see also *Anger*) | Basil, cajeput, cardamom, carrot seed, myrrh, cinnamon (bark, leaf), citronella, grapefruit, | Geranium, helichrysum, hyssop, may |

| | | |
|---|---|---|
| | lemon, lemongrass, patchouli, petitgrain, thyme | chang, nutmeg, peppermint, black pepper, pine needle, rosemary, clary sage, tea tree, turmeric |
| **Concentration** | Cajeput, cypress, eucalyptus, hyssop, lemon, lemongrass, niaouli, nutmeg, bitter orange, peppermint, tea tree, thyme | Basil, ginger, juniper berry. myrtle, patchouli, black pepper, petitgrain, rosemary, sandalwood |
| **Courage** | Angelica root, basil, cajeput, fennel, pine needle, turpentine | Ginger, juniper, oregano, rosemary, clary sage, tea tree |
| **Depression** | Basil, bergamot, chamomile(s), chaste tree, cinnamon, clove bud, frankincense, grapefruit, helichrysum, hyssop, jasmine, lavender, mandarin, marjoram, may chang, melissa (lemon balm), neroli, nutmeg, bitter orange, palmarosa, patchouli, peppermint, petitgrain, rose Otto, clary sage, sandalwood, thyme, ylang ylang | Cardamom, cypress, fennel, lemon, lemongrass, oregano, pine |
| **Disconnection** | Cedarwood Atlas, cinnamon (leaf, bark), fennel, ginger, juniper berry, myrrh, rose, rosemary, vetivert | Cajeput, caraway, cypress, frankincense, grapefruit, hyssop, niaouli, petitgrain, black pepper, pine needle, spikenard, thyme |

| | | |
|---|---|---|
| **Dizziness** | Caraway, pine | Frankincense, lavender, rose, grapefruit, tea tree, turpentine |
| **Fatigue / Exhaustion** | Angelica root, basil, caraway, cardamom, citronella, clove bud, coriander, eucalyptus, frankincense, geranium, ginger, grapefruit, helichrysum, hyssop, juniper berry, lemongrass, may chang, neroli, palmarosa, patchouli, peppermint, pine, rosemary, clary sage | Bergamot, carrot seed, cajeput, cinnamon, lemon, myrrh, bitter orange, black pepper, petitgrain, rose, tea tree, turmeric, turpentine, vetivert |
| **Fear** | Chamomile(s), cypress, fennel, frankincense, geranium, jasmine, juniper berry, melissa, myrtle, patchouli, peppermint, rose Otto, spikenard, valerian, vetivert, ylang ylang | Galbanum, mandarin, bitter orange, clary sage, sandalwood, tea tree |
| **Grief and bereavement (loss)** (see also *Moving on*) | Cypress, frankincense, hyssop, lavender, marjoram, melissa (lemon balm), myrtle, spikenard, rose | Cedarwood, grapefruit, bitter orange |
| **Insomnia** | Angelica root, basil, bergamot, chamomile(s), coriander, geranium, juniper berry, lavender, mandarin, marjoram, may chang, neroli, petitgrain, spikenard, valerian, vetivert, ylang ylang | Carrot seed, cedarwood, cypress, frankincense, helichrysum, mandarin, patchouli peppermint |

| | | |
|---|---|---|
| **Memory** | Clove bud, coriander, cypress, ginger, juniper berry, may chang, melissa (lemon balm), peppermint, rosemary, thyme | Basil, cajeput, bitter orange, petitgrain, pine, tea tree |
| **Moving on** | Cajeput, carrot seed, cypress, eucalyptus, frankincense, helichrysum, black pepper | Grapefruit, myrrh, thyme |
| **Panic attacks** | Chamomile Roman, frankincense, geranium, jasmine, juniper berry, lavender, mandarin, marjoram, melissa (lemon balm), myrrh, patchouli, peppermint, rose, spikenard, vetivert, ylang ylang | Benzoin, caraway, cedarwood, chaste tree, cypress, fennel, bitter orange, neroli, palmarosa, sandalwood, turmeric, valerian |
| **Restorative (revitalising, reviving)** | Basil, bergamot, cajeput, caraway, cardamom. carrot seed, lemon, myrrh, niaouli, peppermint, pine, rosemary, tea tree, turpentine | Clove bud, coriander, eucalyptus, ginger, grapefruit, galbanum, juniper berry, bitter orange |
| **Sedative (calming)** | Angelica root, benzoin, bergamot, cedarwood, chamomile(s), frankincense, lavender, mandarin, marjoram, myrtle, rose, clary sage, sandalwood, spikenard, valerian vetivert | Carrot seed, cypress, geranium, grapefruit, patchouli, palmarosa |
| **Shock / Trauma** | Coriander, frankincense, helichrysum, lavender, marjoram, melissa (lemon balm), neroli, rose, tea tree, ylang ylang | Cajeput, caraway, cedarwood, chamomile roman, cypress, juniper berry, myrrh, peppermint, vetivert, valerian |

| | | |
|---|---|---|
| **Stimulant (tonic)** | Angelica root, cajeput, caraway, clove bud, coriander, lemon, may chang, black pepper, pine, tea tree | Eucalyptus, fennel, ginger, neroli, rose, peppermint |
| **Unwanted thoughts** | Chamomile Roman, cypress, frankincense, lemon, bitter orange, peppermint, sandalwood, pine, tea tree | Carrot seed, citronella, juniper berry, petitgrain rosemary, thyme |

## 20. The psycho-emotional qualities of sixty essential oils

The letters below are applied as symbols to indicate cautions and safety considerations for each of the essential oils listed below. Remember, I do not advocate the internal ingestion of essential oils.  See Methods of Use and Application in the following chapter.

A    Potential dermal irritant, especially when the essential oil is oxidised or old; use fresh and appropriately stored essential oil; do not use on sensitive, damaged, traumatised or diseased skin; do not take internally.

B    Photo toxic; if applied to skin, avoid exposure to sunlight for at least twelve hours and keep the area covered.

C    Avoid during pregnancy, while breastfeeding or during menstruation.

D    Some risk of interaction with certain drugs or medication.

E    Sometimes adulterated - check the authenticity and integrity of the oil with your supplier; use with caution when applying to skin.

Once you have identified essential oils that fit your requirement, you can then refer to the *Essential Oil Scent Profiles*, and *Scent Groups charts in Appendix Two* for more details about each oil's perfume qualities and blending compatibility.

### Angelica Root *Angelica archangelica*   A B C

Eases nervous tension and fatigue; eases insomnia; eases feelings of anxiety; eases migraines and headaches; eases stress-related conditions; promotes feelings of balance and strength; eases 'heartache' and instils a sense of courage. Tonic to the nervous system.

### Basil *Ocimum basilicum*   A C

Aids clarity of thought; strengthens memory; uplifts mood and emotion; eases feelings of anxiety, depression and low mood, and agitation; relieves insomnia and mental and emotional fatigue (encourages emotional strength); relieves premenstrual tension; eases stress and stress-related conditions; encourages intuition.

### Benzoin *Styrax benzoin*   A E

Relieves nervous tension; sedative; warming.

### Bergamot *Citrus bergamia*   B

Balances mood and emotion; allays frustration; refreshing; sedative; uplifting; eases feelings of anxiety, depression and low mood; eases feelings of apathy; relieves insomnia; eases stress and stress-related conditions.

### Cajeput *Melaleuca cajeputi*   A C E

Aids concentration and focus, clears and stimulates the mind and thoughts; eases apathy and low mood; bracing; strengthens the spirit; awakening; helps one find courage in finding new pathways and managing change.

### Caraway *Carum carvi*   A C

Stimulating; tonic to nerves; warming to emotions; replenishes lost energy; eases fatigue; eases mental strain and stress; eases irritability and intolerance; relieves dizziness and vertigo.

**Cardamom** *Elettaria cardamomum*    A E

Uplifting, refreshing, restorative and invigorating (especially during recovery from illness); relieves mental fatigue, nervous tension and exhaustion; eases depression.

**Carrot seed** *Daucus carota*   C

Sedative, relaxant; revitalising; nervous system sedative; eases mental and emotional exhaustion; provides mental clarity; eases anxiety, apathy, and inability to 'move on'.

**Cedarwood Atlas** *Cedrus atlantica*   C

Sedative, calming, balancing and grounding; instils feelings of peace and sense of connection; aids meditation; eases feelings of agitation, anger, sense of disconnectedness and nervous tension; eases feelings of nervousness and hypertension; eases feelings of a 'broken heart'; eases stress and stress-relation conditions.

**Chamomile Roman and German** *Chamaemelum nobile*  A E / *Matricaria recutita* A D E

Mental sedative (calms an active mind); emotional sedative; nervous system sedative; eases mood swings; calms fear, impatience, irritability, intolerance, hyperactivity, hypersensitivity; eases agitation, anger, anxiety, depression and low mood; eases panic attacks; eases solar plexus tension; eases stress and stress-related conditions; eases headache and migraine; aids sleep.

**Chaste Tree** *Vitex agnus castus*    C

Eases anxiety and depression; calms erratic moods; eases premenstrual tension

**Cinnamon leaf** *Cinnamomum verum, C. zeylanicum* A C D E

Stimulant; strengthening; arouses senses and creativity; eases feelings of mental and emotional weakness, tension and nervous exhaustion; eases sense of isolation and emotional coldness; eases fear, depression and low mood; eases stress and stress-related conditions.

**Citronella** *Cymbopogon winterianus, C. nardus*  A E

Clearing and uplifting; eases feelings of depression, fatigue, headaches, migraine, and neuralgia; eases stress and stress-related conditions.

**Clove bud** *Syzugium aromaticum, Eugenia caryophyllus*   A D

Stimulant; stimulates mental functions; uplifting; aphrodisiac (impotence, frigidity); aids memory and recall; eases depression and low mood, mental and emotional fatigue; eases lethargy; eases headaches, tension, stress and stress-related conditions.

**Coriander** *Coriandrum sativum*   A D E

Mental stimulant (gentle); aids and restores memory and recall; eases headaches and migraine; eases debility, nervous exhaustion and insomnia.

**Cypress** *Cupressus sempervirens*   E

Sedative; uplifting; regulates autonomic nervous system; eases lack of concentration, aids focus and memory recall; eases confusion and indecision; eases anger, anxiety, depression and low mood, fear, grief, bereavement (loss), impatience, uncontrollable crying, dwelling on unpleasant events; shifts inability to move on and feelings of being 'stuck'; eases nervous tension and premenstrual tension; balancing; eases stress and stress-related conditions.

**Eucalyptus** *Eucalyptus globulus*

Bracing; clears head and eases over-thinking; aids concentration; assists in moving on from past trauma; eases fatigue and debility; soothes neuralgia and headaches.

**Fennel** *Foeniculum vulgare*  C D E

Gives courage and instils a sense of protection; tonic to nerves; eases nervous tension, stress and stress-related conditions.

**Frankincense** *Boswellia carteri, B. neglecta, B. sacra*

Sedative; supports meditation and finding inner tranquillity; balances mood swings; eases inability to move on, and dwelling on unpleasant events; helps in letting go of unwanted thoughts and memories, resentment and disappointment, sadness and despair; eases anger, anxiety, depression and low mood, fear, grief and bereavement; eases end-of-life agitation; eases panic attacks (calms and relaxes breathing), and nervous tension; eases confusion and indecision; calms hyperactivity; eases stress and stress-related conditions.

### Galbanum *Ferula gummosa*   A

Balancing, both sedative and stimulant; uplifting; calming; tonic; restorative to nerves; eases anxiety, depression and low mood; calms erratic moods; eases premenstrual tension and nervous tension and menopausal symptoms; eases stress and stress-related conditions.

### Geranium *Pelargonium graveolens, P. x asperum*   E

Balancing; both sedative and stimulant; uplifting; balances nerves and solar plexus; eases nervous tension and fatigue; eases anger, anxiety, depression and low mood; eases feelings of fear; endocrine stimulant (hormone-like); eases headaches and insomnia (low dose); eases premenstrual tension and menopausal symptoms; eases stress and stress-related conditions.

### Ginger *Zingiber officinale*

Stimulating, yet grounding; offers psychic and emotional protection; aids memory and recall; warms cold emotions; eases debility, emotional pain, nervous exhaustion and tiredness.

### Grapefruit *Citrus x paradisi*   E

Uplifting; supports withdrawal from addiction (especially when combined with vetivert and/or frankincense); improves sense of self-confidence; eases feelings of depression and low mood; relieves headache; eases nervous exhaustion, emotional fatigue, stress and stress-related conditions.

### Helichrysum (Immortelle) *Helichrysum angustifolium, H. italicum*

Aid's ability to let go of the past and move on; eases feelings of depression and low mood, mental and emotional debility, burnout and nervous exhaustion; relieves headaches (especially those caused by liver congestion); relieves shock; eases stress and stress-related conditions; good for meditation.

**Hyssop** *Hyssop officinalis*   C

Aids concentration and focus; eases anxiety, depression and low mood, mental and emotional fatigue; eases feelings of grief; eases nervous tension; eases stress and stress-related conditions; instils a sense of spirituality.

**Jasmine** *Jasminum grandiflorum*   A E

Euphoric; uplifts mood and emotions; improves sense of self-confidence; eases feelings of anxiety, depression and low mood; eases feelings of fear; eases nervous tension, stress and stress-related conditions; good for meditation.

**Juniper berry** *Juniperus communis*   A

Dispels negative energy; strengthening; uplifting; aids memory; quells confusion and indecision; eases feelings of anxiety, fear, hypersensitivity, nervous tension and fatigue; eases stress, stress-related headaches and other stress-related conditions; balances mood and emotion; good to use in preparation for formal meditation.

**Lavender English and Spike** *Lavandula angustifolia, L. latifolia*   E

Central nervous system sedative (sedative at low dose, stimulant at high dose); eases panic attacks; eases feelings of agitation, anger, anxiety, depression and low mood, grief, bereavement and loss, feelings of hopelessness, irritability, intolerance and impatience, nervous tension and premenstrual tension; eases insomnia; eases feelings of shock and solar plexus tension; eases stress and stress-related conditions.

**Lemon** *Citrus limonum*   A E

Mental stimulant; clears thoughts and aids concentration; uplifts and eases feelings of anxiety; aids a sense of balance and control; eases feelings of apathy; eases stress and stress-related conditions.

**Lemongrass** *Cymbopogon citratus, C. flexuosus*   A D

Sedative; awakens; eases feelings of apathy and mental and emotional fatigue, irritability and intolerance; helps with lack of concentration and nervous exhaustion; eases stress, stress-related headaches and other stress related conditions.

**Mandarin** *Citrus reticulata*

Awakens; brings out the inner child; sedative; uplifting; eases anxiety, depression and low mood; quells hyperactivity (while orange can encourage hyperactivity, mandarin is calming); alleviates insomnia; eases nervous tension and panic attacks (combine with frankincense) and restlessness; eases premenstrual tension, stress and stress-related tension.

**Sweet Marjoram** *Origanum marjorana, Marjorana hortensis*  C

Stimulates the parasympathetic nervous system; reassuring and steadying; calms hyperactivity; soothes an overactive mind; eases anxiety, depression and low mood, feelings of grief and heartache, irritability and agitation, nervous tension, hypertension; aids sense of self confidence; eases insomnia, headaches and migraine; eases stress and stress-related conditions.

**May Chang** *Litsea cubeba*  A D

Stimulant; uplifting; eases feelings of anxiety, depression and low mood; eases feelings of fatigue and lethargy; eases memory loss and insomnia.

**Melissa (Lemon balm)** *Melisa officnialis*  A E

Raises the spirits; uplifting; tonic; strengthens memory; calming; eases feelings of anxiety, depression and low mood, fear and shock, grief, bereavement and loss; eases feelings of nervousness and hypertension; eases insomnia.

**Myrrh** *Commiphora myrrha, C. erythraea*  A C E

Both sedative and stimulant; calming; revitalising; regulates and calms breathing; grounding; eases apathy and warms emotional coldness; brings emotions to the surface; good for meditation.

**Myrtle** *Myrtus communis*  D

Sedative; neuro-balancing; soothes anger; eases feelings of despair, fear, grief, bereavement and loss; eases distraction and insomnia.

**Neroli (Orange blossom)** *Citrus x aurantium var. amara*  E

Relaxing; tranquillising (low dose), stimulating (high dose); instils a sense of peace; calms the nervous system and eases nervous tension and premenstrual tension; eases feelings of anxiety, depression and low mood; eases feelings of agitation, emotional shock and upset, sadness and disappointment; eases fatigue and insomnia; encourages feelings of self-confidence; eases stress and stress-related conditions.

### Niaouli *Melaleuca quinquenervia*

Reviving; aids concentration; clears head; eases depression and low mood (especially when caused by illness or infection).

### Nutmeg *Myrista frangrans*   C

Mental stimulant; warming and euphoric (hallucinogenic in large dose); eases depression and low mood; eases feelings of emotional coldness; intensifies dreams.

### Bitter Orange *Citrus aurantium var. amara*   B

Uplifting and refreshing; stimulant; energises; supports enthusiasm; supports sympathetic nervous system; aids mental clarity and concentration; eases anxiety, depression and low mood; instils a sense of balance and control; eases insomnia, stress and stress-related conditions.

### Oregano *Origanum vulgaris*   A

Stimulating, uplifting and reviving; eases feelings of depression; encourages feelings of steadfastness and courage.

### Palmarosa *Cymbogopogon martini*

Grounding and uplifting; eases anxiety, depression and low mood; eases fatigue, headache and migraine; eases agitation, stress and stress related conditions.

### Patchouli *Pogostemon cablin*   E

Sedative at low dose, stimulant at high dose; regulates and calms breathing; eases feelings of anxiety, panic attacks, nervous tension and exhaustion; eases confusion and indecision, agitation and apathy; eases premenstrual tension, stress and stress related conditions; supports meditation and a sense of spirituality.

**Black Pepper** *Piper nigrum*

Mental stimulant; aids alertness; eases cold feelings and adds warmth to indifference; eases transition and life changes; grounding.

**Peppermint** *Mentha x piperita*   A  E

Eases breathing; refreshing and invigorating; awakening; sedative and calming in low dose; eases panic attacks; eases depression and low mood; calms racing thoughts and mental chatter; improves concentration; aids memory loss; eases mental fatigue and exhaustion; eases nervous tension; eases stress and stress related conditions.

**Petitgrain** *Citrus aurantium var. amara*   E

Uplifting and calming; restores mental clarity; aids focus; nervous system sedative; eases anxiety, depression and low mood, apathy and nervous tension, anger and agitation; eases hyperactivity, insomnia, mental and nervous exhaustion; eases premenstrual tension, stress and stress-related conditions.

**Pine Needle (Scotch)** *Pinus sylvestris*   E

Bracing; refreshes and stimulates a tired mind; clears head; eases debility; eases and sense of hopelessness, fatigue and nervous exhaustion; eases stress and stress-related conditions

**Rosemary** *Salvia Rosmarinus*   A

Restorative; stimulating; tonic; enlivens the brain and clears head; aids memory; aphrodisiac; eases depression and low mood; eases debility, lethargy, mental fatigue and nervous exhaustion; eases headaches and migraine; aids in opening the throat chakra and finding your voice.

**Rose Otto** *Rosa x damascene, R. centifolia*   E   **Absolute**  A

Balancing; stimulant and high dose, sedative at low dose; hypnotic; aphrodisiac; eases nervous tension and panic attacks; eases anxiety, depression (especially postnatal) and low mood, grief, bereavement and sense of loss; eases feelings of fear, paranoia, agitation, anger and jealousy; eases mood swings (especially hormonal); eases feelings of resentment and disappointment, sadness and despair; eases premenstrual tension and menopausal symptoms; eases feelings of shock; eases stress and stress-related conditions.

### Clary Sage *Salvia sclarea*   C

Sedative; mildly intoxicating (potentiated by alcohol); euphoric; aphrodisiac; bracing during difficult times; eases anxiety, depression and low mood; relieves nervous tension and fatigue; eases migraine and headache.

### Sandalwood *Santalum album, S. spicatum*   D

Sedative; aphrodisiac; tonic; calms and harmonises the mind; calms racing thoughts, mental chatter and mental clutter; eases agitation, anxiety, depression and low mood; eases end-of-life agitation; eases insomnia, feelings of stress and stress-related conditions; aids meditation.

### Spikenard *Nardostachys jatamansii, N. grandiflora*

Balances sympathetic nervous system with parasympathetic nervous system (tonic to the sympathetic nervous system, regulates the parasympathetic nervous system); eases panic attacks and feelings of fear and dread; calms restlessness; inspires a sense of peace and spirituality; eases anxiety, depression and low mood; eases feelings of heartache, bereavement and loss; grounds feelings of hatred; calms hyperactivity, hysteria, impatience, restlessness and insomnia; eases headache and migraine; eases menopausal symptoms, stress and stress-related symptoms; aids meditation.

### Tea Tree *Melaleuca alternifolia*   A

Stimulating; revitalising; aids concentration and focus; clears and stimulates the mind; eases feelings of apathy and nervous exhaustion; eases feelings of shock.

### Thyme *Thymus vulgaris, T. zygis*   A

Tonic; uplifting; calming; aphrodisiac; aids concentration and memory; aids in letting go of anger and frustration; encourages release of mental blocks; strengthens and supports higher heart and throat chakra; eases depression and low mood; relieves insomnia; eases headache; eases stress and stress-related conditions; grounding (thyme linalool).

**Turmeric** *Curcuma longa*

Grounding yet stimulating; gently dispels feelings of stagnation; gently uplifts spirits; warming and comforting; gently brightens mood, emotion; eases feelings of anxiety, debility and nervous exhaustion.

**Turpentine** (Longleaf Pine) *Pinus palustris*   A

Bracing; clears head, and dispels 'negative energy'; eases debility, fatigue, and nervous exhaustion; eases neuralgia; eases feelings of disconnection; relieves stress-related conditions.

**Valerian** *Valeriana officinalis, V. jatamansi*

Tranquilising; hypnotic; calming; grounding and earthing; eases feelings of anxiety and tension; eases insomnia, nervousness, restlessness and agitation; eases stress and stress-related conditions.

**Vetivert** *Vetiveria zizanioides*

Encourages feelings of tranquillity; sedative to the nervous system; grounding; reduces symptoms of withdrawal when coming off pharmaceutical drugs (especially tranquillisers); eases feelings of anxiety, depression and low mood, confusion, indecision, mental debility and exhaustion; eases restlessness and agitation, hyperactivity, hypersensitivity, irritability, intolerance, impatience; eases premenstrual tension, stress and stress-related conditions; eases insomnia.

**Yarrow** *Achillea millefolium*   D

Uplifts spirit and mood; supports intuition; eases tension; eases stress and stress-related conditions.

**Ylang Ylang** *Cananga odorata*   A

Relaxes the central nervous system; aphrodisiac; euphoric; uplifts mood; stimulant; eases anxiety, depression and low mood; eases nervous tension; eases feelings of panic, fear, and shock; calms anger and rage; eases insomnia; eases stress and stress-related conditions.

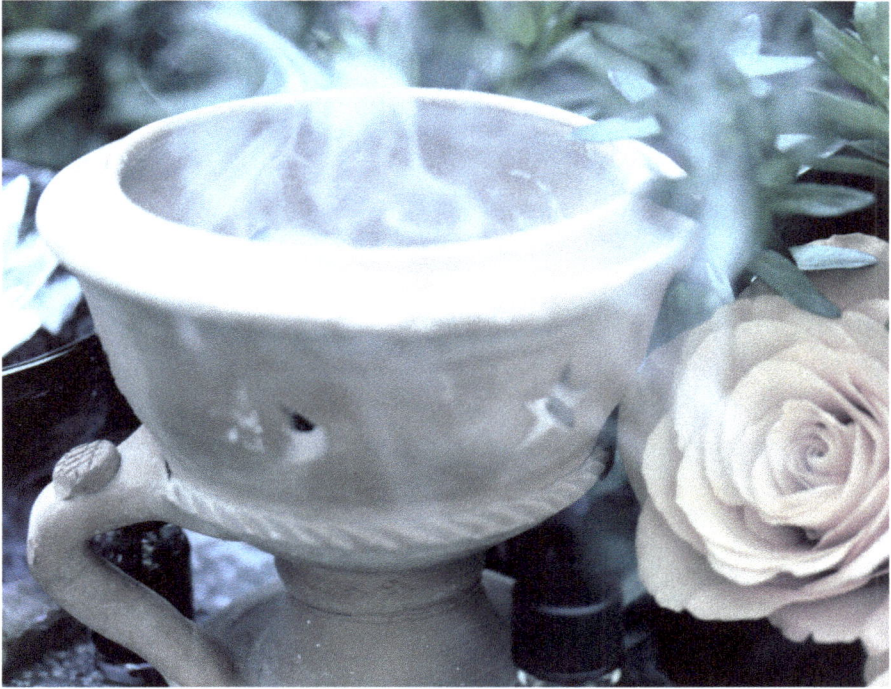

## 21. Methods of use and application

### Candle-lit room diffuser

- Add water to the bowl. Add six to eight drops of a single essential oil or an essential oil blend. Light candle. Replenish as necessary.

- Candle-lit diffusers with deep water bowls are preferable (to avoid rapid drying out). Keep a small jug of water at hand to replenish, and do not allow the water bowl to dry out.

- Do not leave unattended – ensure the candle is extinguished before leaving unattended. Place the diffuser in a safe and stable position, where it cannot be knocked over (candles and essential oils are a fire risk) or touched by children or pets.

- Do not diffuse essential oils close to people's heads. If using a diffuser in a communal area, such as an office or waiting room, always check that other people like the oils you are diffusing and/or that they do not have respiratory problems that may be irritated by essential oil molecules.

### Electric fan or steam diffusers

These usually come with instructions regarding appropriate operation and use. Add six to eight drops of an essential oil or essential oil blend. Replenish as necessary.

Rather than leaving the diffuser on constantly, use in short 'bursts' at chosen convenient times. Remember, the sense of smell soon becomes saturated; the brain stops acknowledging smells after a short period of time, even though they may still be present (leaving and returning to a room, the odour is re-acknowledged; this may be a good indication of whether the essential oils need replenishing).

Just as with candle-lit diffusers, above, do not diffuse essential oils close to people's heads. If using a diffuser in a communal area, such as an office or waiting room, always check that other people like the oils you are diffusing and/or that they do not have respiratory problems that may be irritated by essential oil molecules.

## Baths

Fill bath with water, then, just before getting in, add six drops of essential oil or an essential oil blend dispersed in twenty millilitres of vegetable oil. Do not use essential oils neat in the bath. To maximize benefit, close windows and doors.

Remember, vegetable oil makes the bath slippery. Do not leave children unattended in a bath.

Although wetting and soaking the skin with warm water may assist some epidermal absorption of essential oil molecules, it also increases the risk of skin irritation. Also, hot or warm baths tend to encourage perspiration (excretion) rather than absorption through sweat glands. Also, essential oils tend to remain on the surface of water and will evaporate quite quickly into the atmosphere. Absorption, therefore, is more likely to occur as a result of inhaling essential oil-infused steam vapours, rather than via epidermis (skin) absorption.

Also, water itself is very 'drying' to the skin, and when combined with neat essential oils, this drying effect is increased. Essential oils, therefore, should be dispensed in an oily or fatty carrier medium (emollient) such as grapeseed or olive oil; thus, an oily barrier is created that may prevent essential oil irritation and reduce the 'drying' effect of water to the skin.

A better option is to diffuse the essential oil(s) into the atmosphere, or to apply the essential oils topically in a non-perfumed lotion, cream or vegetable oil after bathing, while the skin is hydrated and refreshed after a bath; thus, also slowing down water loss through evaporation after bathing and aiding moisturisation and suppleness of the dermis through creating a gentle barrier and improving absorption of the essential oils.

# CAUTION: ESSENTIAL OILS THAT
# SHOULD NOT BE USED IN THE BATH

Basil, cinnamon, clove, peppermint, thyme, citrus oils or lemon-scented oils.

### Steam Inhalation

You will need: a kettle (or pan), water, bowl, tissues, essential oils and a large towel. Before commencing, ensure that your equipment is placed in a safe position, away from pets and children and on a stable surface.

Heat the water to boiling point. Very carefully pour boiled water from the kettle (or pan) into the bowl (preferably heat proof ceramic, glass or pottery – do not use plastic bowls). Allow the water to cool slightly (essential oils will vaporise too rapidly otherwise). Add two to four drops of your selected essential oil or blend of essential oils to the water (replace essential oil bottle lids immediately).

Cover your head and the bowl with the large towel to contain the rising essential oil infused steam vapours – CLOSE YOUR EYES. Breathe vapours through your nose, exhale through your mouth, for a few minutes. Remove towel ('come up for air'). Replenish water and essential oils if necessary and repeat exercise two or three times.

Stop immediately if you experience any irritation, or feel dizzy. Essential oils will irritate the mucous membrane to a certain degree; use moderately and do not exceed the above dose. Caution must be applied if the recipient has sensitivities, asthma or epilepsy (always check a particular oil is not contraindicated and, if safe to use, only use half the above dose – one to two drops of essential oils).

### Aroma Sticks (Nasal Inhalers)

These can be purchased from most aromatherapy equipment suppliers. Dismantle the tube-like inhaler to remove the wadding roll inside. Add 2 to 6 drops of your selected essential oil, or essential oil blend, to the wadding. Replace the essential oil-infused wadding within the tube, secure the protective cap then screw on the protective cover.

To apply, remove the cover, hold the tube to your nose, and inhale through each nostril as required. Replace the protective cover immediately after use.

## Resin Burner

This method is reserved for resins rather than essential oils; for example, frankincense resin or myrrh resin. A small, flat piece of charcoal held firmly with long-handled pincers or tweezers, is lit. Once the charcoal sparks, it will rapidly heat. Still using the tweezers, the smouldering charcoal is placed within the bowl of the container and a small piece of resin is placed on top of it. As the charcoal heats the resin, the resin begins to smoke as it melts and disintegrates; the essential oil is carried within the smoke that infuses into the surrounding atmosphere.

Do not leave the resin burner unattended once lit. Place the container in a safe position where it cannot be accidently knocked over or touched by children or pets. Always ensure that the charcoal and resin have burned out. Once finished with, douse with water to extinguish if still burning.

## 22. Guidelines for measuring essential oils

Measuring essential oils quantities is complicated, especially given variation in dropper size and oil viscocity, which renders absolutely accurate measurement impossible as the quantity of essential oil released per drop varies. However, in the interest of safety, essential oil quantities do need careful consideration. The measurements set out in the guide below are based on average droplet sizes.

Risk of sensitivity or irritation increases where large amounts of oil are applied to small areas of skin: applying six drops of essential oil in a carrier medium to the whole body through massage will have negligible irritant effect, yet the same quantity of oil applied to a small area of skin can be irritant, particularly in sensitive areas such as the face, or under arms if used as deodorants, and so on. If you experience any skin or respiratory tract irritation (itching, redness, rashes, swelling, breathing difficulty) stop applying the essential oil or the blend of essential oils immediately.

Remember, use essential oils within their stipulated use-by date (found on the bottle or packaging).

Use no more than one or two drops of essential oils in a carrier medium on localised areas of skin. Keep this in mind when making first aid ointments or face creams or lotions. When making face creams or ointments for repeated regular use, make up small quantities that can be used up quickly and frequently refreshed; reduce the amounts of essential oils included; change the essential oil selection and/or blend from time to time; and have 'no essential oil' breaks in between use.

**Safe Measurements**

As a guide:

- A five-millilitre bottle of essential oil contains approximately one hundred drops of essential oil

- A ten-millilitre bottle of essential oils contains approximately two hundred drops of essential oil

- Maximum amount of essential oil per twenty-four-hour period: six to ten drops (healthy adult – see below)

- Apply for two to three weeks only, followed by one week's abstinence, and change essential oil(s) selection regularly

   Note: Carrier medium means or refers to vegetable oils, non-perfumed creams, lotions, ointments and gels

- One drop of essential oil in five millilitres of carrier medium - one per cent blend

- Two-and-a-half drops of essential oil in five millilitres of carrier medium - two-and-a-half percent blend (round up or down – two or three drops)

• Five drops of essential oil in five millilitres of carrier medium - five per cent blend

**Appropriate quantities guidelines**

Reduce amounts for children and babies over three months old, and for those who are frail or have sensitivities.  Please note, I do not advocate the use of essential oils for infants under three years old, but include advice here to ensure careful considered use.

Use maximum dilution (one drop of essential oil in twenty millilitres of vegetable oil or non-perfumed cream or lotion) for babies between three months and thirty-six months old, and **do not** use herbaceous, spicy, citrus oils, highly perfumed oils, or citrus-like oils such as lemongrass or citronella, and always ensure the genuine purity of your essential oil before applying – that is, one hundred per cent pure unadulterated, preferably organic, essential oil purchased from a reputable supplier who provides relevant safety information.

Also, use increased dilution for those who are frail or very elderly and those with sensitivities, allergies, eczema, asthma, and for facial blends.  For example:

• One drop of essential oil in ten millilitres of carrier medium - half a percent blend

• Two drops of essential oil in twenty millilitres of carrier medium - half a percent blend

• One drop of essential oil in twenty millilitres of carrier medium - a quarter percent blend (babies and toddlers three months to twenty-four months – as above, do not use herbaceous, spicy or citrus oils)

**Normal amount for general and adult use guidelines**

- Two-and-a-half drops of essential oil in five millilitres of carrier medium - two-and-a-half percent blend (rounded up or down)

- Five drops of essential oil in ten millilitres of carrier medium - two-and-a-half percent blend

**Exceptional amount for acute, short-term occasional use. Avoid or reduce the use of known irritant essential oils.**

- Five drops of essential oil in five millilitres of carrier medium - five percent blend

- Ten drops of essential oil in ten millilitres of carrier medium - five percent blend

- One drop of essential oil in twenty millilitres of carrier medium - a quarter percent blend (babies and toddlers three months to thirty-six months – as above, do not use herbaceous, spicy or citrus oils)

## 23. Essential Oil Safety

Applied appropriately, there is no doubt that essential oils are highly beneficial psycho-emotional, antimicrobial, skin healing, pleasant 'scentual' agents. However, it is important to remember they are highly concentrated, volatile, organic phyto-chemicals, with propensity to be very drying and irritant to skin and mucous membranes (as previously mentioned), and as such, require careful handling. Because they are volatile, essential oils rapidly evaporate, oxidise and degrade, especially if they are not stored correctly, which increases their propensity to cause irritation and sensitivity. Degradation of an essential oil occurs naturally over time, but is detrimentally exacerbated in the presence of heat and UV light, and when the essential oil is exposed to oxygen, which can result in the oil becoming toxic, sensitising, and corrosive, or, especially in terms of their therapeutic qualities, inert. To slow these reactions down and to preserve their optimum quality, essential oils are best stored in a cool dark place, such as a fridge, in non-corrosible brown or blue glass, or aluminium, UV protected bottles or containers, with dropper dispensing caps and tightly secured lids.

## Storage and care guidelines

- Only purchase essential oils from reputable suppliers whose oils are ethically and ecologically appropriately sourced, extracted and handled, and who will provide safety data information and details about their chemical composition and source (plant and botanical species, location of growth, and so on).

- Only purchase essential oils stored in amber or dark blue glass bottles with 'dropper top' lids (to ensure careful measurement, to prevent spillage or accidental ingestion, and to slow down oxidisation). Some suppliers place the essential oil-filled glass bottle in an additional canister, or sleeve, that prevents light infiltration. This ensures the essential oil is protected from over-exposure to UV light.

- Check the sell-by date before use and make a note of the date of purchase (essential oils have a limited shelf life). Generally, essential oils will last for up to two years if unopened, and one year once opened (citrus oils, such as mandarin or lemon, for up to six months once opened). Pine oils, including turpentine, and other oils with high terpene content, like citrus oils, oxidise rapidly. Some oils oxidise slowly, for example, sandalwood, vetivert, myrrh and rose and their integrity may linger for some time past their sell-by-date (once past the usual sell-by date, these oils are best not used on skin, but may make lovely perfumes in small amounts, a little dab on clothes).

- Discard small amounts of essential oil left in a bottle or container, unless the essential oil is used up rapidly from the moment of first opening the bottle. NB: do not flush residue or old unused essential oils down the sink or toilet as their oxidised chemicals can be harmful/toxic to fish and the local aquatic micro-biome.

- Replace lids immediately after use (to slow down oxidisation).

- Never 'top-up' a bottle of essential oil with more essential oil once opened for use.

- Store in a cool dark place, away from sources of heat and direct sunlight (preferably a fridge – some oils, such as rose Otto, however, will solidify when very cold, but will return to a liquid state at room temperature), to protect the oil from rapid oxidisation (exacerbated by light, heat, and atmospheric oxygen).

## Safe application guidelines

- Check out the safety data of an essential oil before using or applying it; not all essential oils are safe or appropriate to use in all circumstances or conditions, for example, during pregnancy, during the course of the application of certain medications or treatments, and so on. (*See Healing with Essential Oils,* pages 181 to 316)

- Do not apply essential oils neat to the skin (always dilute in a vegetable oil, non-perfumed lotion or cream – for example, one or two drops of essential oil to five millilitres of vegetable oil). Undiluted dermal application of essential oils can lead to irritation and sensitisation. Lavender and tea tree essential oils are the exception to this rule (often used as a first aid remedy for insect stings, minor burns or skin abrasions, or mild skin infections), but repeated long term topical application of these oils is not advisable due to the risk of sensitisation.

- Do not swallow or take essential oils internally (see Accidents and Reactions below) unless professionally prescribed by an appropriately trained herbalist, healthcare practitioner, chemist, or doctor.

- To avoid sensitisation, do not use the same essential oil or blend of essential oils repeatedly; take breaks from use (every two or three weeks), and vary the essential oils you use if applying them over a long period. Also, use limited quantities (no more than six drops per day). Essential oils are highly concentrated; very small amounts are very effective.

- Always ensure that the essential oils you select are compatible with your requirement and are otherwise not contra-indicated; especially significant if you are taking prescribed medication, such as painkillers (for example, codeine or other opiate derivatives) or blood thinning medication, and so on.

- Wipe up spillages immediately (essential oils will dissolve / damage polystyrene, plastic, varnish, paint, polished and laminated surfaces).

**Babies and children: guidelines**

- Do not use essential oils for babies under three months old.

- I also do not recommend use of essential oils for infants aged between three months and thirty-six months. If applied during this age range, they must be used in extreme moderation (one drop of essential oil in twenty millilitres of carrier medium – vegetable oil, non-perfumed cream or lotion). DO NOT use herbaceous, spice, citrus oils (with the exception of mandarin), citral or lemon-scented oils (such as, lemongrass or citronella), or highly perfumed oils (such as, ylang ylang). The skin and vital organs of babies are still developing, especially the organs of elimination; essential oils are highly concentrated and can cause a toxic reaction or organ damage in babies and young children. Also, an infant's immune system, particularly their adaptive immune system, does not begin to fully function until they are around three or four years old, and does not become fully functional until after the first ten years of life; a child's immune system acquires strength and resilience through 'practice', that is, through coming into contact with and combating and resisting minor infections – thus setting up a template for future combat. Over use of antibiotics, anti-microbial, disinfecting and sterilising products, including inappropriate application of essential oils, during this phase, may detrimentally hinder this vital ground laying process.

- NEVER, to reiterate, apply undiluted essential oils to a child, infants or baby's skin and NEVER add undiluted essential oils to their bath.

- NEVER use essential oils for internal consumption.

- Do not put drops of essential oils directly onto pillows due to the risk of eye contact.

- Keep essential oils out of the reach of children (good suppliers will provide child-proof lids if requested) and keep away from pets.

- Essential oils are best diffused into the environment, away from an infant's head space to avoid irritation of the airways, perhaps to soothe restlessness, and/or to aid sleep.

## Accidents and reactions guidelines

- Accidental ingestion: DO NOT INDUCE VOMITING. Drink full fat milk. Seek medical advice immediately. Keep the bottle the essential oil was stored in for identification (the label should display the Latin name, batch no., sell-by date etc., and the bottle will have traces of the oil).

- Eyes: Essential oils can be transferred from your fingers to your eyes (always wash your hands after using or handling essential oils). If NEAT essential oil enters your eyes IMMEDIATELY flush with vegetable oil or full fat milk, then rinse thoroughly with clean, warm water. Sometimes diluted essential oils enter the eyes during steam inhalation, bathing or showering. If this happens immediately flush eyes with clean warm water. In either case, seek medical advice IMMEDIATELY if irritation or stinging persists after flushing your eye(s).

- Skin reaction: Apply vegetable oil to dilute the essential oil on the skin, then thoroughly wash the area with non-perfumed soap (liquid soap if possible) and rinse with warm water to remove any trace of soap and the essential oil. Dry the area thoroughly and apply a non-perfumed base cream (vegetable oil or even butter if nothing else is available) to soothe irritation if appropriate.

(Godfrey 2022, 2020, 2019)

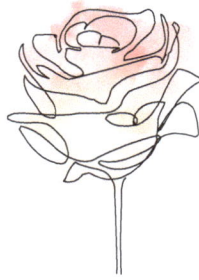

My books, *Healing with Essential Oils, Essential Oils for the Whole Body,* and *Essential Oils for Mindfulness and Meditation,* along with this book, collectively provide comprehensive information and detail about safe and effective application of essential oils.  For example, *Essential Oils for the Whole Body, Chapter Three, Safe Practice and Contraindication; and Healing with Essential Oils, Chapter Four, Essential Oil Chemistry: A brief Introduction to the Science of Plant Constituents.* These books also include insightful background information and detail about the role of essential oils within the plant, related botany, various methods of extraction, related organic chemistry, how to blend effective therapeutic and aesthetic remedies and perfumes, how the oils are absorbed and excreted by the body, and in-depth profiles of fifty-eight individual essential oils (including all the essential oils mentioned in this book), and much more - along with this book, your quintessential essential oil 'go to' guides.

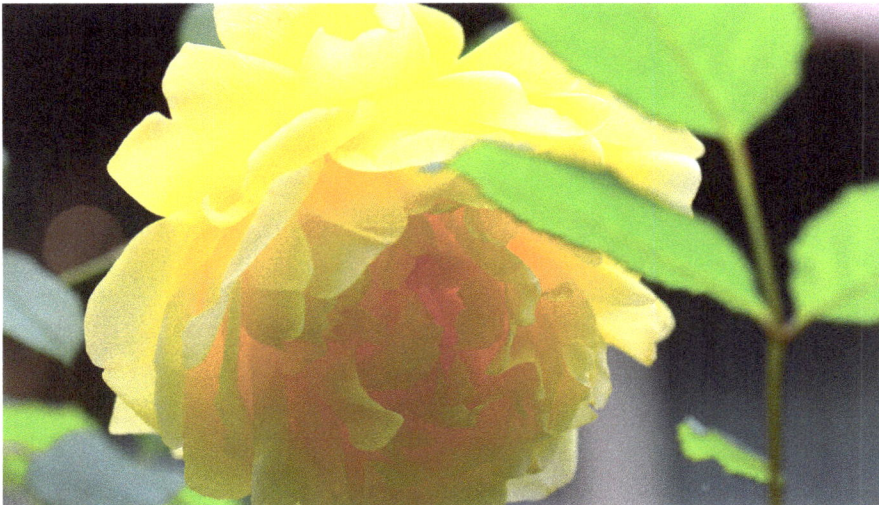

# Signs, symptoms and causes of anxiety and depression

## Signs and Symptoms of Anxiety

**Psychological**
A sense of dread or fearing the worst.
Being easily distracted
Depersonalisation (a type of disassociation from your mind or body, or like you are a character that you are watching in a film)
Derealisation (another type of disassociation where you feel disconnected from the world around you, or that the world is not real)
Feeling constantly 'on edge'
Feeling like the world is speeding up or slowing down
Feeling like other people can see you are anxious and are looking at you
Feeling like you cannot stop worrying, or that bad things will happen to you if you stop worrying
Feeling tense, nervous or unable to relax
Impatience
Irritability
Low mood and depression
Restlessness
Rumination – thinking a lot about bad experiences, or thinking over a situation again and again
Wanting lots of reassurance from other people or worrying that people are angry or upset with you
Worrying a lot about things that might happen in the future
Worrying about anxiety itself, for example, worrying about when panic attacks might happen
Worrying that you are losing touch with reality

**Physical**
A churning feeling in your stomach.
Backache
Changes in your sex drive
Diarrhoea
Difficulty falling or staying asleep
Drowsiness and tiredness

## Signs and Symptoms of Depression

**Psychological**
A sense of unreality
Agitated
Angry or frustrated over minor things
Anxiety
Cognitive dysfunction and difficulty concentrating
Difficulty speaking clearly or making decisions
Difficulty remembering things
Feeling empty and numb
Feeling guilty
Feelings of worthlessness or hopelessness
Feeling down, upset or tearful
Finding no pleasure in life or things you usually enjoy
Hopeless and despairing
Isolated and unable to relate to other people
Irritability
Lack of enthusiasm
Loss of interest in hobbies or activities
Moving very slowly
No self-confidence or self-esteem
Restlessness
Thoughts of suicide

**Physical**
Appetite changes
Digestive issues
Fatigue and feeling tired all the time, lethargy
Headaches
Head feels heavy
Limbs feel heavy

Dry mouth
Excessive sweating
Excessive thirst
Faster or shallow breathing
Feeling light-headed or dizzy
Frequent urinating
Grinding your teeth
Headache
Hot flushes
Irregular heartbeat (palpitations)
Muscular aches and pains
Nausea
Painful or missed periods
Pins and needles
Shortness of breath
Stomach ache
Unable to sit still

**Causes**
Adrenal dysfunction
Asthma
Chronic disease
Current life situation
Depressive disorders
Diabetes
Drugs and medication side effects
Financial insecurity
Gut health – microbiome imbalance
Heart disease / cardiac issues
Housing insecurity, homelessness, poor living conditions
Hyperthyroidism
Hypoglycaemia
Inflammatory disorders or diseases
Irritable Bowel Syndrome (IBS)
Lack of oxygen
Nutrient deficiency
Negative self-talk (cause and symptom)
Over-thinking (cause and symptom)
Past or childhood experiences
Poor diet
Physical and mental health conditions
Sensitivity to certain foods and chemicals
Stress (including financial, medical issues, social, political, unpredictable or uncertain world events, such as pandemics, pressure at work, other stressful life events)
Trauma, shock, disturbance
Watching and listening to mainstream news
Work and job insecurity

Persistent aches or pains
Sexual dysfunction, loss of interest
Sleep disturbance
Weight loss or weight gain

**Causes**
Alcohol and drugs
Current life situation
Drugs and medication side effects
Family history, genetics
Financial insecurity or worry
Giving birth - post natal depression
Gut health – microbiome imbalance
Head injury
Heart disease
Hormonal imbalance
Housing insecurity, homelessness, poor living conditions
Illness and medical conditions
Lack of sunlight
Lack of exercise
Loneliness
Negative self-talk (cause and symptom)
Neurotransmitter (serotonin, norepinephrine, dopamine) imbalance
Nutrition deficiency
Poor diet (processed foods, excessive sugar and refined fats, oils and carbohydrates).
Stress (financial, medical issues, social, political, unpredictable or uncertain world events, such as pandemics, pressure at work, other stressful events)
Toxicity from mould or metals
Trauma, shock, disturbance
Underactive thyroid
Unresolved emotional problems
Watching and listening to mainstream news
Work and job insecurity

# Health and medical conditions that may cause anxiety or anxiety-like symptoms

- Attention Deficit Hyperactive Disorder (ADHD)

- Chronic pain

- Drug misuse or withdrawal

- Endocrine conditions

- Gastro-intestinal conditions

- Inflammatory conditions

- Metabolic conditions

- Misuse of or withdrawal from alcohol

- Neurological disorders: strokes, epilepsy, multiple sclerosis, traumatic brain injury, dementia

- Panic disorder

- Parathyroid and adrenal gland conditions

- Phobias

- Post-Traumatic Stress Disorder (PTSD)

- Respiratory disorders and conditions: for example, chronic obstructive pulmonary disease (COPD), asthma

- Thyroid problems (hyperthyroidism, hypothyroidism)

- Withdrawal from anti-anxiety medication (for example, benzodiazepines)

# Other potential causes of anxiety

- Brain chemistry

- Dehydration

- Environmental factors

- Free floating anxiety (anxiety that cannot be obviously attributed to any specific issue)

- Genetics

- Stress

- Traumatic events

- Vitamin deficiency

# Traits of the
# Highly Sensitive Person

- Affected by other people's moods
- Annoyed or frustrated when asked to do too many things at once
- Appreciates and enjoys delicate fine scents, tastes, sounds and works of art
- Aware of subtleties and nuances within the surrounding environment
- Avoids violent movies and TV programmes or dramas
- Avoids upsetting or overwhelming situations
- Becomes unpleasantly aroused when a lot is going on locally
- Being very hungry creates a reaction, disrupting concentration or mood
- Conscientious
- Deeply moved by art or music
- Dislikes being observed while performing; becomes nervous or shaky
- Easily overwhelmed by things like bright lights, strong smells, coarse fabrics, or alarms or sirens close by
- Has a rich, complex inner life
- Made uncomfortable by loud noises
- Need to withdraw during busy days, perhaps into bed or into a darkened room or a place of privacy and solace and relief from stimulation
- Observant of other people's discomfwort in an environment and tend to know what needs to be done to make it more comfortable (like changing the lighting or seating)
- Rattled or annoyed when having a lot to do in a short amount of time
- Seen as being sensitive or shy by parents and teachers as a child
- Sensitivity to the effects of caffeine
- Startles easily
- Tend to be very sensitive to pain
- Tries hard to avoid making mistakes or to forget things
- Unsettled by too much change

(Aron 1999)

APPENDIX TWO

# Aligning seasons and subtle dynamics and essential oil blending compatibility

## Subtle Characteristics:
## Ancient Chinese yin and yang, and essential oils

| Yang | Yang / Yin | Yin |
|---|---|---|
| Basil (French) | Angelica root | Benzoin |
| Cinnamon | Bergamot | Cajeput |
| Clove bud | Caraway | Chamomile German |
| Grapefruit | Cardamom | Chaste tree |
| Lemongrass | Carrot seed | Cypress |
| May Chang | Cedarwood | Fennel seed |
| Melissa (Lemon balm) | Chamomile Roman | Geranium |
| Nutmeg | Citronella | Helichrysum / Immortelle |
| Pepper, black | Coriander | Hyssop |
| Rosemary | Eucalyptus globulus | Juniper berry |
| Tea tree (some indication) | Frankincense | Lemon |
| Turmeric | Galbanum | Niaouli |
| | Ginger | Rose Otto |
| | Jasmine | Sage, clary |
| | Lavender | Sandalwood |
| | Mandarin | Tea tree |
| | Marjoram | Vetivert |
| | Myrrh | Yarrow |
| | Myrtle | |
| | Neroli (Orange blossom) | |
| | Orange bitter/sour | |
| | Oregano | |
| | Palmarosa | |
| | Patchouli | |
| | Peppermint | |
| | Petitgrain (Orange leaf) | |
| | Pine needle | |
| | Rose absolute | |
| | Spikenard | |
| | Thyme linalool | |
| | Turmeric | |
| | Turpentine | |
| | Valerian | |
| | Ylang Ylang | |

# Chakras and essential oils:

| 1<br>Base Red | 2<br>Sacral Orange | 3<br>Solar Plexus Yellow | 4<br>Heart Pink / Green |
|---|---|---|---|
| Benzoin | Angelica root | Angelica root | Basil |
| Helichrysum/Immortelle | Benzoin | Basil | Bergamot |
| Lemongrass | Caraway | Bergamot | Cajeput |
| May Chang | Carrot seed | Cajeput | Chamomile German |
| Myrrh | Cedarwood Atlas | Caraway | Chamomile Roman |
| Neroli absolute | Chaste tree | Cardamom | Coriander |
| Orange bitter / sour | Cinnamon | Carrot seed | Cypress |
| Rose absolute | Citronella | Cedarwood Atlas | Eucalyptus globulus |
| Thyme, thymol (red) | Clove bud | Chamomile Roman | Frankincense |
| Valerian | Coriander | Chaste tree | Galbanum |
| Vetivert | Ginger | Cinnamon | Geranium |
| | Helichrysum/Immortelle | Citronella | Ginger |
| | Jasmine | Clove bud | Grapefruit |
| | Lemongrass | Coriander | Hyssop |
| | Marjoram | Cypress | Juniper berry |
| | May Chang | Eucalyptus globulus | Lavender |
| | Melissa | Fennel | Lemon |
| | Myrrh | Frankincense | Mandarin |
| | Myrtle | Galbanum | Niaouli |
| | Neroli absolute | Geranium | Orange, sweet |
| | Nutmeg | Ginger | Palmarosa |
| | Orange bitter / sour | Grapefruit | Pepper, black |
| | Palmarosa | Helichrysum/Immortelle | Peppermint |
| | Patchouli | Hyssop | Rose otto |
| | Pine needle, Scotch | Jasmine | Rose absolute |
| | Rose absolute | Juniper berry | Sage, clary |
| | Sandalwood | Lavender | Sandalwood |
| | Spikenard | Lemon | Spikenard |
| | Thyme, linalool | Lemongrass | Tea tree |
| | Turmeric | Marjoram, sweet | Thyme, linalool |
| | Valerian | May Chang | Valerian |
| | Vetivert | Melissa | Yarrow |
| | Ylang Ylang | Myrrh | |
| | | Myrtle | |
| | | Neroli (Orange blossom) | |
| | | Niaouli | |
| | | Nutmeg | **Thymus Turquoise** |
| | | Orange bitter / sour | **(Blue-green)** |
| | | Palmarosa | |
| | | Pepper, black | *Situated between heart* |
| | | Peppermint | *and throat chakra* |
| | | Petitgrain (orange leaf) | |
| | | Pine needle, Scotch | Clove bud |
| | | Rose Otto | Eucalyptus globulus |
| | | Rosemary | Thyme |
| | | Sage, clary | |
| | | Sandalwood | |
| | | Tea tree | |
| | | Thyme, linalool | |
| | | Turmeric | |
| | | Turpentine | |
| | | Ylang Ylang | |

| 5 Throat Blue | 6 Third Eye / Brow Violet | 7 Crown White / Violet |
|---|---|---|
| Chamomile German | Lavender | Basil |
| Chamomile Roman | Patchouli | Frankincense |
| Lavender | | Lavender |
| Pepper, black | | |
| Rosemary | | |
| Spikenard | | |
| Yarrow | | |

# Body Clock (circadian rhythm) and elemental characteristics

| Dominant time of day | Body Clock activity | Element | Hippocrates / Avicenna Humour | Characteristic qualities | Associated body structures | Zodiacal Relationship | Associated personality traits | Ayurvedic Dosha |
|---|---|---|---|---|---|---|---|---|
| 9pm – 12am | Melatonin production building; core body temperature dropping; time to go to sleep. 'Larks' (early risers) tend to go to bed earlier, 'owls' (late risers) tend to go to bed later. | Earth / Metal / Ether | Atrabilious (Melancholic) | Earthy and gross (dense), cold, dry, thick, black and sour. Autumn | Spleen, blood; bones | Taurus Virgo Capricorn | Pessimistic, reserved, despondent, unsociable, quiet. Moody, anxious, irritable, restless, rigid, Sober. | Kapha |
| 12am – 3am | Sleep hormone melatonin peaking; minimum levels of attention and vigilance. Bowel 'closes down' for the night – a reason not to eat large or heavy meals in the evening. | | | | | | | | |
| 3am – 6am | Body soundly asleep; minimum core body temperature; severe asthma attacks more common. | Water | Phlegmatic (Serous) | Watery, cold, moist, white Winter | Fluids, tissues and nutrition; circulation, joints | Cancer Pisces Scorpio | Controlled, reliable, even tempered, patient, calm. Passive, careful, thoughtful, relaxed, peaceful. | Pitta / Kapha |
| 6am – 9am | Optimum time to wake up; heart attacks more likely; blood vessels are stiffer and more rigid, blood is thicker and stickier; blood pressure is at its peak; men – testosterone peak. Good time to drink water. | | | | | | | | |
| 9am – 12pm | Mind most alert; stress hormone (cortisol) levels peak, boosting alertness and the brain's short-term memory capacity. | Air / Wood | Sanguineous | Hot, moist, sweet, red Spring | Respiration and circulation | Leo Aries Sagittarius | Easygoing, lively, carefree, leadership. Talkative, outgoing, sociable, pleasure-seeking, responsive. | Vatta |
| 12pm – 3pm | Biological siesta; increased gastric activity; post lunchtime dip in alertness (surge in road accidents). Bad time to drink alcohol – causes more drowsiness than at other times during the day. | | | | | | | | |
| 3pm – 6pm | Best time to exercise; best lung and cardiovascular performance; muscles 6% stronger, core body temperature rising to its peak. | Fire | Bilious (Choleric) | Hot and dry, yellow or red, Bitter Summer | Liver, gall bladder; digestion | Gemini Aquarius Libra | Changeable, impulsive, optimistic, active, a 'doer', leader. Touchy, aggressive, short-tempered, irritable, restless, excitable, dominant. | Pitta |
| 6pm – 9pm | Poor time to eat a big meal (light meals preferable; the body alters the way it handles food during the evening; liver handles alcohol better; intuitive thinking is better. | | | | | | | | |

# Ayurveda and the qualities of the three doshas Vatta, Pitta, and Kapha

| Dosha | Attributed energetic qualities | | The five associated sub-doshas, their physical location, dynamic governance and foods to balance |
|---|---|---|---|
| Vatta | Spring<br>Air / Ether / Wood<br>Mobile / Dynamic<br>Respiration<br>Circulation<br>Locomotion<br>Movement<br>Elimination<br>The whole nervous system<br>Speech | Creativity<br>Enthusiasm<br>Dry<br>Light<br>Cold<br>Rough<br>Subtle<br>Mobile<br>Clear<br>Dispersing<br>Astringent / bitter | **Prana:** brain, head, throat, lungs and heart; inhalation and the senses through perception.<br><br>**Udana:** navel, nose, throat and lungs; speech, self-expression, effort, enthusiasm, strength and vitality<br><br>**Vyana:** skin, heart, permeates through the whole body; circulation, heart rhythm, locomotion<br><br>**Samana:** stomach and small intestine<br><br>**Apana:** between the navel and the anus<br><br>*Foods to balance Vatta: dark leafy greens, vegetables, raw fruits, legumes, herbs and spices* |
| Pitta | Summer<br>Fire / Water<br>Energetic / Transformative<br>Digestion<br>Metabolism<br>Vision<br>Complexion<br>Body temperature<br>Intelligence<br>Discrimination<br>Courage | Cheerfulness<br>Oily<br>Sharp<br>Hot<br>Penetrating<br>Light<br>Mobile<br>Liquid<br>Fleshy<br>Sour / pungent | **Pachaka:** lower stomach, duodenum and small intestine; digestion of food as its broken down into nutrients and waste, emulsifying fats<br><br>**Ranjaka:** liver, gall bladder and spleen; formation of red blood cells and synthesis of hemoglobin, gives color to blood and stools<br><br>**Alochak:** eyes; visual perception<br><br>**Sadhaka:** head, brain and heart; emotions, memory, intelligence, 'digestion of thoughts'<br><br>**Bharajaka:** skin; luster and complexion, sweat and sebaceous glands, temperature and skin pigmentation<br><br>*Foods to balance Pitta: sour fruits, yogurts, fermented foods, chilli peppers, garlic, herbs and spices* |
| Kapha | Autumn / winter<br>Earth / Metal / Water<br>Anabolic processes<br>Lubrication<br>Fluid secretion<br>Fluid balances<br>Potency<br>Patience<br>Heaviness<br>Understanding | Compassion<br>Heaviness / heavy<br>Slow<br>Cold<br>Oily / Slimy / Smooth<br>Dense / Soft<br>Static / Stable<br>Cloudy / Sticky<br>Hard / Gross<br>Sweet / Salty | **Kledaka:** upper stomach; moistening and liquifying of food in the initial stages of digestion<br><br>**Avalambhka:** chest, heart and lungs; lubrication of the heart and lungs, strength to the back, chest and heart<br><br>**Tarpaka:** head, sinuses and cerebrospinal fluid; calmness, happiness and stability, nourishment of the sense and motor organs<br><br>**Bodhaka:** tongue, mouth and throat; perception of taste, lubricating and moistening of food<br><br>**Shleshaka:** joints; lubrication of all joints<br><br>*Foods to balance Kapha: fruits, grains, natural sugar, milk, natural salts and sea vegetables* |

# Chinese Medicine body clock elements, seasonal conditions and essential oils

| Time of day/ night | Element / Direction | Season / Emotion | Body structure / organ | Activity | Essential Oils |
|---|---|---|---|---|---|
| 7am – 9am | Earth (Ground)<br>West<br>Yin Yang<br>High energy | Changing seasons<br>Autumn<br>Damp<br>Love | Stomach | Breakfast<br>Walk<br>Concentration | Angelica root (yang, yin)<br>Benzoin (yin)<br>Bergamot (yang, yin)<br>Cardamom (yin, yang)<br>Carrot Seed (yin, yang)<br>Caraway (yang, yin)<br>Cedarwood (yang, yin)<br>Chamomile German (yin)<br>Cinnamon (yang)<br>Coriander (yang, yin)<br>Fennel (yin, yang)<br>Frankincense (yin, yang)<br>Galbanum (yang, yin)<br>Ginger (yang, yin)<br>Helichrysum (yin)<br>Lemon (yin)<br>Mandarin (yin, yang)<br>Marjoram (yin, yang)<br>Myrrh (yang, yin)<br>Myrtle (yin, yang)<br>Neroli (yang, yin)<br>Nutmeg (yang)<br>Orange bitter (yang, yin)<br>Palmarosa (yang, yin)<br>Patchouli (yin, yang)<br>Peppermint (dried) (yang, yin)<br>Petitgrain (yin, yang)<br>Pine Needle (yin, yang)<br>Sage, Clary (yin)<br>Sandalwood (yin, yang)<br>Spikenard (yang, yin)<br>Thyme (yin, yang)<br>Turmeric (yang)<br>Valerian (yin, yang)<br>Vetivert (yin)<br>Ylang Ylang (yin, yang) |
| 9am – 11am | Earth (Ground/Spirit)<br>West<br>Yin Yang<br>High energy | Changing seasons<br>Autumn<br>Damp<br>Love | Spleen | Food converted to chi<br>Clear thinking | |
| 11am – 1pm | Fire<br>South<br>Yang<br>High energy | Summer<br>Hot<br>Happiness | Heart | Lunch<br>Blood circulation<br>High energy | Basil (yang)<br>Bergamot (yang, yin)<br>Citronella (yin, yang)<br>Ginger (yang, yin)<br>Jasmine (yin, yang)<br>Lemongrass (yang)<br>May chang (yang)<br>Nutmeg (yang)<br>Rosemary (yang)<br>Orange bitter (yang, yin)<br>Peppermint (fresh) (yang, yin) |
| 1pm – 3pm | Fire<br>South<br>Yang<br>Resting energy | Summer<br>Hot<br>Happiness | Small Intestine | Sort and absorb food<br>Low energy<br>Rest / sleep | Angelica root (yang, yin)<br>Caraway (yang, yin)<br>Cinnamon (yang)<br>Coriander (yang, yin)<br>Black pepper (High altitude) (yang)<br>Lemon balm (Melissa) (yang)<br>Mandarin (yang, yin)<br>Neroli (yang, yin)<br>Palmarosa (yang, yin)<br>Spikenard (yang, yin)<br>Turmeric (yang) |
| 3pm – 5pm | Water<br>North<br>Yin<br>Passive energy | Winter<br>Cold<br>Fear / scared | Bladder | Energy restored after rest and food absorption<br>Liquid waste released<br>Work / study | Cajeput (yin)<br>Cypress (yin)<br>Geranium (yin)<br>Ginger (yang, yin)<br>Jasmine (yin, yang)<br>Juniper (yin)<br>Lemon (yin)<br>Rose otto (yin)<br>Sandalwood (yin, yang)<br>Thyme (yin, yang) |
| 5pm – 7pm | Water<br>North<br>Yin<br>Passive energy | Winter<br>Cold<br>Fear / scared | Kidney | Eat<br>Store nutrients<br>Build bone marrow | Cedarwood (yang, yin)<br>Chamomiles (yin, yang)<br>Black pepper (low altitude) (yang)<br>Grapefruit (yang)<br>Myrtle (yin, yang)<br>Orange sweet (yin)<br>Yarrow (yang) |

| Time | Element / Direction / Polarity / Energy | Season / Climate / Emotion | Organ | Functions | Essential oils |
|---|---|---|---|---|---|
| 7pm – 9pm | Fire, South, Yang, Calm energy | Late summer, Hot, Happiness, Boundaries | Pericardium | Protection, Self-care, Relaxation, Light reading | Bergamot (yang, yin), Frankincense (yin, yang), Lemon balm (melissa) (yang), Lemongrass (yang), Spikenard (yang, yin), Rose otto (yin) |
| 9pm – 11pm | Fire, South, Yang, Calm energy | Late summer, Hot, Happiness, Boundaries | Triple burner | Endocrine and metabolic balance, Prepare for sleep | Lemongrass (yang), Peppermint (yang, yin), Petitgrain (yin, yang), Spikenard (yang, yin), Valarian (yin, yang), Ylang Ylang (yin, yang) |
| 11pm – 1am | Wood, East, Yin Yang, Resting energy | Spring, Wind / Air, Anger | Gall Bladder | Sleep, Bile release, Cellular repair, Build blood cells | Angelica seed, Cardamon (yin, yang), Chamomile Roman (yin), Orange bitter (yang, yin), Grapefruit (yang), Lavender (yin, yang), Lemon balm (melissa) (yang) |
| 1am – 3am | Wood, East, Yin Yang, Resting energy | Spring, Wind / Air, Anger | Liver | Deep sleep, Blood detox, Rest and recovery, Planning | Cardamon (yin, yang) (Recovery from bad dreams), Cypress (yin), Fennel (yin), Myrrh (yang, yin) |
| 3am – 5am | Metal, Ether, Earth (Spirit), Yin, Recuperating energy | Autumn, Dry / cold, Grief and sadness | Lungs | Deep sleep, Lung detox, Dreams, Memory | Pine needle (yin, yang), Sage, Clary Sage (yin), Sandalwood (yin, small yang), Turpentine (yin), Yarrow (yin); Lavender (yin, yang), Myrrh (yang, yin), Niaouli (yin), Rose otto (yin) |
| 5am – 7am | Metal, Ether, Earth (Spirit), Yin, Recuperating energy | Autumn, Dry / cold, Grief and sadness | Large Intestines | Wake up, Release bowel, Meditate | Cajeput (yin), Cypress (yin), Frankincense (yin, yang), Galbanum (yang, yin), Geranium (yin) |

# Seasons, direction and ancient wisdom

| Traditional Category | North | North East | East | South East | South | South West | West | North West |
|---|---|---|---|---|---|---|---|---|
| **Season** | Winter | Transition Winter - Spring | Spring | Transition Spring - Summer | Summer | Transition Summer - Autumn | Autumn | Transition Autumn - Winter |
| **Plant cycle** | Resting and Dormant | | Stirring and New Growth | | Blossoming and Flowering | | Ripening, Fruiting, Harvesting | |
| **Element** | Water | | Air / Wood | | Fire | | Earth / Metal | |
| **Humor / Temperament** | Phlegmatic | | Sanguine | | Choleric | | Melancholic | |
| **Quality** | Cold / Moist | Wet | Hot / Moist | Hot | Hot / Dry | Dry | Cold / Dry | Cold |
| **Zodiac** | | Taurus Virgo Capricorn | | Gemini Aquarius Libra | | Leo Aries Sagittarius | | Cancer Pisces Scorpio |
| **Wisdom Relationship** | | Grandfather | | Grandmother | | Great Spirit / Father | | Mother |
| **Celestial** | | Moon | | Rising Sun | | Stars | | Earth |
| **Colour** | White | | Yellow | | Red | | Black | |
| **Nation** | Creeping and crawling nation | | Winged nation | | Green and growing nation | | Four-legged nation | |
| **Insect** | Dragonfly / Spider | | Earthworm | | Honey Bee / Cicada | | Chrysalis / Butterfly | |
| **Animal** | Great White Buffalo / Wolf | | Eagle | | Coyote / Mouse | | Bear | |

| | | | | |
|---|---|---|---|---|
| **Condition / Ancient Wisdom** | Illumination / Teacher / Guidance / Wisdom / Gratitude / Connection between the natural world and spirit (divine) world / Visionary Consciousness / Fulfilling potential | Emerging Life / Planting / New Beginnings / Expansion of consciousness / New Thought / Transformation / Birth / Inspiration / Fertilizing / Reconciling the past / Contemplation / Listening | Creative / Formation of New Dreams and Creations / Youth / Action / Alchemy / Manifestation / Sacred Union / Co-creation / Purpose and sacred practice / Social cooperation / Abundance / Nourishment | Authentic Soul alignment with divine intuition and unique purpose / Brings Spirit into Matter / Maturity / Adult / Empathy / Soulful metamorphosis / Wounded healer / Feelings / Heart / Higher good<br><br>The elements metal and ether are also associated with higher love |
| **Associated Essential Oils** | Bergamot<br>Cedarwood<br>Grapefruit<br>Frankincense<br>Lemon<br>Mandarin<br>Myrrh<br>Orange, bitter / sour<br>Pepper, black – low altitude<br>Turmeric<br>Vetivert<br>Ylang Ylang<br><br>*Supporting Essential Oils*<br>Melissa (Lemon Balm)<br>Rose Otto | Angelica seed<br>Cypress<br>Geranium<br>Neroli (Orange leaf)<br>Pepper, black – high altitude<br>Rose Otto<br>Spikenard<br>Tea Tree<br>Thyme<br>Valarian<br><br>*Supporting Essential Oils*<br>Grapefruit<br>Palmarosa<br>Lemon<br>Pine needle<br>Juniper berry | Angelica root<br>Benzoin<br>Carrot seed<br>Chamomile's<br>Chaste Tree<br>Hysop<br>Jasmine<br>Lavender<br>Melissa (Lemon balm)<br>Myrrh<br>Peppermint<br>Pettigrain (Orange leaf)<br>Pine needle<br>Nutmeg<br>Rosemary<br>Sage, Clary<br>Turpentine<br>Yarrow<br><br>*Supporting Essential Oils*<br>Bergamot<br>Grapefruit<br>Lemon<br>Lime<br>Mandarin<br>Neroli (Orange blossom)<br>Rose Otto | Angelica root<br>Cardamom<br>Coriander seed<br>Cypress<br>Fennel seed<br>Frankincense<br>Grapefruit<br>Juniper Berry<br>Neroli (Orange blossom)<br>Marjoram<br>May Chang<br>Peppermint (dried)<br>Spikenard<br>Turmeric<br>Valarian<br><br>*Supporting Essential Oils*<br>Lemon<br>Orange bitter / sour<br>Palmarosa<br>Valarian<br>Vetivert |

In addition to Water, Air/Wood, Fire, Earth/Metal, Ether represents 'above' and 'below', esoteric wisdom, higher love, the chakras, honouring life's journey, surrender and preparing to 'fly' (Star-Wolf and Cariad-Barrett 2013)

# Native Indian seasons and moons

| North | North East | East | South East | South | South West | West | North West |
|---|---|---|---|---|---|---|---|
| Winter | Winter – Spring | Spring | Spring – Summer | Summer | Summer – Autumn | Autumn | Autumn – Winter |
|  | Grandfather |  | Grandmother |  | Great Spirit / Father |  | Mother |
|  | Moon |  | Rising sun |  | Stars |  | Earth |
| December | January / February | March | April / May | June | July / August | September | October / November |

| Month | Moon | Hunting and gathering (Adapt foods and harvest to local geographical seasons) |
|---|---|---|
| January | Spirit moon. Wolf moon. | Spear fish through ice. Fish. |
| February | Bear moon. Snow moon | Check traps. Rabbit. |
| March | Snow crust moon. Worm moon. Sap and sugar moon. | Sugar Bush Camp. Maple syrup. |
| April | Sugar moon. Pink moon. Moon of red grass appearing | Birchbark (medicine, scroll). Wild leeks. |
| May | Sucker moon. Flower moon. Budding moon. Planting moon. | Pick strawberries. Strawberry. |
| June | Blossom moon. Strawberry moon. Green corn moon | June Berry Bush. June Berry. |
| July | Berry moon. Buck moon. Salmon moon. Raspberry moon. Thunder moon | Pick berry. Plum, raspberry, blackberry. |
| August | Ricing moon. Sturgeon moon. Grain moon. | Wild ricing. Wild rice. Blueberry. |
| September | Changing leaves moon. Harvest moon (harvest), Equinox moon. | Chokeberry. Wild potato. |
| October | Full corn moon. Harvest moon (harvest) | Deer. Cranberry. Corn. |
| November | Falling leaves moon. Drying rice moon. Hunters moon (harvest) | Deer. Cranberry. |
| December | Freezing moon. Frost moon. Beaver moon. Big spirit moon (13th moon) | Hunting grouse. Sharp-tailed grouse. |

# Essential oil-bearing plants, optimal harvest times and related seasons

| | North · December WINTER | North East · January/February Winter/Spring | East · March SPRING | South East · April/May Spring/Summer | South · June SUMMER | South West · July/August Summer/Autumn | West · September AUTUMN | North West · October/November Autumn/Winter |
|---|---|---|---|---|---|---|---|---|
| Angelica root | | | | | | Angelica root/seed | Angelica root/seed | Angelica root |
| Basil | | | | | | Basil | Basil | |
| Benzoin | | | | | Benzoin | Benzoin | | |
| Bergamot | Bergamot | Bergamot | Bergamot | | | | | Bergamot |
| Cajeput | | | | | | Cajeput | Cajeput | |
| Caraway seed | | | | | | Caraway seed | Caraway seed | |
| Cardamom | | | | | | | Cardamom | Cardamom |
| Carrot seed | | | | | | Carrot seed | | |
| Cedarwood | | Cedarwood | | | | | | |
| Chamomile's | | | | | Chamomile's | Chamomile's | | |
| Chaste Tree | | | | | Chaste Tree | Chaste Tree | | |
| Cinnamon Bark/Leaves | Cinnamon Bark/Leaves | Cinnamon Bark/Leaves | Cinnamon Bark/Leaves | Cinnamon Bark/Leaves | Cinnamon Bark/Leaves | Cinnamon Bark/Leaves | Cinnamon Bark/Leaves | Cinnamon Bark/Leaves |
| Citronella | | Citronella | | Citronella | | Citronella | Citronella | Citronella |
| Clove bud | *India, Brazil* Clove bud | *India, Brazil, Tanzania* Clove bud | *Tanzania* Clove bud | *Indonesia* Clove bud | *Indonesia* Clove bud | *Indonesia* Clove bud | *Indonesia* Clove bud | |
| Coriander seed | | | | | | Coriander seed | Coriander seed | |
| Cypress | Cypress | Cypress | Cypress | Cypress | | | | Cypress |
| Eucalyptus | | Eucalyptus | | Eucalyptus | | Eucalyptus | | Eucalyptus |
| Fennel seeds | | | | | | Fennel seeds | Fennel seeds | |

| Essential Oil | North — December WINTER | North East — January/February Winter/Spring | East — March SPRING | South East — April/May Spring/Summer | South — June SUMMER | South West — July/August Summer/Autumn | West — September AUTUMN | North West — October/November Autumn/Winter |
|---|---|---|---|---|---|---|---|---|
| Frankincense | Frankincense | Frankincense | Frankincense | Frankincense | Frankincense | | | Frankincense |
| Galbanum resin | | | | | | Galbanum resin | Galbanum resin | |
| Geranium | | | Geranium | Geranium | | Geranium | Geranium | |
| Ginger | Ginger | | | | | Ginger | Ginger | Ginger |
| Grapefruit | Grapefruit | | | Grapefruit | Grapefruit | Grapefruit | | Grapefruit |
| Helichrysum | | | | | Helichrysum | Helichrysum | Helichrysum | |
| Hyssop | | | | | Hyssop | Hyssop | | |
| Jasmine | | | | | Jasmine | Jasmine | | |
| Juniper berry | | | | | | | Juniper berry | Juniper berry |
| Lavender | | | | | Lavender | Lavender | | |
| Lemon | Lemon (esp. winter) | Lemon (esp. winter) | Lemon | Lemon | Lemon | Lemon | Lemon | Lemon |
| Lemongrass | Lemongrass | Lemongrass | | Lemongrass | Lemongrass | Lemongrass | Lemongrass | Lemongrass |
| Mandarin | Mandarin | Mandarin | | | | | | Mandarin |
| Marjoram | | | | | | Marjoram | Marjoram | |
| May Chang | | | | | | May Chang | May Chang | |
| Lemon Balm/Melissa | | | | | | Lemon Balm/Melissa | | |
| Myrrh | Myrrh | Myrrh | | | Myrrh | Myrrh | | |
| Myrtle | | | | Myrtle | Myrtle | Myrtle | Myrtle | Myrtle |
| Neroli | | | | Neroli | | | | Neroli |
| Niaouli | Niaouli | Niaouli | Niaouli | | | | Niaouli | Niaouli |
| Nutmeg | | | | | Nutmeg | Nutmeg | | |

| Column 1 | Column 2 | Column 3 | Column 4 | Column 5 | Column 6 | Column 7 | Column 8 |
|---|---|---|---|---|---|---|---|
| Orange, bitter | | Orange, bitter | | Orange, bitter | Orange, bitter | Orange, bitter | Orange, bitter |
| | | | | | Orange, sweet | Orange, sweet | Orange, sweet |
| Palmarosa | | Oregano | | Oregano | | Palmarosa | |
| Patchouli | | Palmarosa | | Palmarosa | | Patchouli | |
| | | Patchouli | | Patchouli | | | Pepper, black low alt |
| | Peppermint (fresh) | | Peppermint (fresh) | Pepper, black high alt. | | Pepper, black low alt | |
| | | Lavender | Lavender | | | | |
| | | Petitgrain | Petitgrain | Petitgrain | | | |
| | | Pine Needle | Pine Needle | | | | |
| | | Rosemary | Rosemary | | | | |
| | | | Rose absolute | Rose | | | |
| | | Sage, Clary | Sage, Clary | Sage, Clary | | | |
| Sandalwood | Sandalwood | Sandalwood | | | Sandalwood | Sandalwood | Sandalwood |
| Spikenard | | | | | Spikenard | | |
| | | Tea Tree | | | Tea Tree | | |
| | | | Thyme | Thyme | Thyme | | Turmeric |
| Turmeric | | | | | | | |
| Turpentine | Turpentine | Turpentine | Turpentine | Turpentine | | | |
| | Valarian | | | | Valarian | | |
| Vetiver (subtropic/med) | Vetiver (sub tropic) | Vetiver (sub tropic) | | Vetiver (sub tropic) | Vetiver (sub trop/med) | Vetiver (sub trop/med) | Vetiver (sub trop/med) |
| | | Yarrow | Yarrow | | | | |
| | | | | | Ylang Ylang | Ylang Ylang | Ylang Ylang |

**AUTMN**
**Specific Essential Oils**

Angelica root
Cardamom
Coriander seed
Cypress
Fennel seed
Frankincense
Grapefruit
Juniper Berry
Marjoram
May Chang
Neroli
Peppermint (dried)
Spikenard
Turmeric
Valarian

**SUMMER**
**Specific Essential Oils**

Angelica root
Benzoin
Carrot seed
Chamomile's
Chaste Tree
Hyssop
Jasmine
Lavender
Lemon Balm (Melissa)
Myrrh
Oregano
Peppermint
Petitgrain
Pine Needle
Nutmeg
Rosemary
Sage, Clary
Yarrow

**SPRING**
**Specific Essential Oils**

Cypress
Geranium
Neroli
Pepper, Black – high altitude
Rose
Spikenard
Tea Tree
Thyme
Valarian

**WINTER**
**Specific Essential Oils**

Bergamot
Cedarwood
Frankincense
Grapefruit
Lemon
Mandarin
Myrrh
Orange
Pepper, Black – low altitude
Turmeric
Vetivert
Ylang Ylang

# Seasons, elements and essential oils

| East / Spring<br>Wood / Air | South / Summer<br>Fire | West / Autumn<br>Earth (Ground) | Earth (Spirit)<br>Metal / Ether | North / Winter<br>Water |
|---|---|---|---|---|
| Angelica seed | Angelica root | Angelica root | Cajeput | Cajeput |
| Cardamon | Basil | Benzoin | Chamomile German | Chamomile German |
| Chamomile Roman | Bergamot | Bergamot | Chaste tree | Chamomile Roman |
| Ginger | Caraway | Caraway | Cypress | Cypress |
| Grapefruit | Cinnamon | Cardamom | Eucalyptus globulus | Cedarwood Atlas |
| Lavender | Citronella | Carrot seed | Fennel | Geranium |
| Lemongrass | Clove bud | Cedarwood Atlas | Frankincense | Ginger |
| Marjoram | Coriander | Cinnamon | Galbanum | Jasmine |
| Melissa (Lemon balm) | Frankincense | Citronella | Geranium | Juniper berry |
| Neroli (Orange blossom) | Ginger | Clove bud | Hyssop | Lemon |
| Orange bitter / sour | Jasmine | Coriander | Lavender | Myrtle |
| Peppermint | Lemongrass | Eucalyptus globulus | Myrrh | Orange sweet |
| Petitgrain | Mandarin | Fennel | Niaouli | Rose Otto |
| Rose absolute | May Chang | Frankincense | Pine needle | Sandalwood |
| Spikenard | Melissa (Lemon balm) | Galbanum | Rose Otto | Thyme, linalool |
| Valerian | Neroli | Ginger | Sage, clary | Vetivert |
| Ylang Ylang | Nutmeg | Helichrysum / Immortelle | Sandalwood | Yarrow |
| | Orange bitter / sour | Lemon | Tea tree (predominantly) | |
| *Supporting Essential Oils* | Oregano | Mandarin | Turpentine | *Supporting Essential Oils* |
| | Palmarosa | Marjoram | Yarrow | |
| Cypress | Pepper, black | Myrrh | | Bergamot |
| Geranium | Rose absolute | Myrtle | *Supporting Essential Oils* | Grapefruit |
| Lemon | Rosemary | Neroli (Orange bitter) | | Frankincense |
| Juniper | Spikenard | Nutmeg | Cardamom | Mandarin |
| Palmarosa | Tea tree | Orange bitter / sour | Coriander seed | Melissa (Lemon Balm) |
| Pepper, Black – high altitude | Thyme thymol (red) | Palmarosa | Grapefruit | Myrrh |
| Pine | Turmeric | Patchouli | Juniper Berry | Pepper, Black – low altitude |
| Tea Tree | | Peppermint | Lemon | Turmeric |
| Thyme | *Supporting Essential Oils* | Petitgrain (Orange leaf) | Neroli | Ylang Ylang |
| Valarian | | Pine needle | Marjoram | |
| | Benzoin | Rose absolute | May Chang | |
| | Carrot seed | Sage, clary | Orange bitter / sour | |
| | Chamomile's | Sandalwood | Palmarosa | |
| | Chaste Tree | Spikenard | Peppermint (dried) | |
| | Hyssop | Thyme linalool | Spikenard | |
| | Lavender | Turmeric | Turmeric | |
| | Myrrh | Valerian | Valarian | |
| | Peppermint | Vetivert | Vetitvert | |
| | Petitgrain (Orange leaf) | Ylang Ylang | | |
| | Pine Needle | | | |
| | Nutmeg | *Supporting Essential Oils* | | |
| | Sage, Clary | | | |
| | Turpentine | Cypress | | |
| | Yarrow | Grapefruit | | |
| | | Juniper Berry | | |
| | | May Chang | | |

# Scent groups

| Amber | Anisic | Balsamic | Citrus / Citral | Herby | Spicy |
|---|---|---|---|---|---|
| Angelica root | Basil<br>Fennel | Benzoin<br>Myrrh<br>Turpentine | Bergamot<br>Citronella<br>Grapefruit<br>Lemon<br>Lemongrass<br>Mandarin<br>May Chang<br>Melissa<br>Orange bitter | Cajeput<br>Caraway<br>Carrot Seed<br>Chamomile(s)<br>Chaste Tree<br>Eucalyptus<br>Helichrysum<br>Hyssop<br>Myrtle<br>Niaouli<br>Oregano<br>Rosemary<br>Clary Sage<br>Thyme<br>Valerian<br>Yarrow | Cardamon<br>Cinnamon bark / leaf<br>Clove bud<br>Coriander<br>Ginger<br>Marjoram<br>Nutmeg<br>Black pepper<br>Tea tree<br>Turmeric |
| **Woody** | **Terpenic** | **Green** | **Floral** | **Minty** | **Earthy** |
| Cedarwood<br>Patchouli<br>Sandalwood<br>Spikenard<br>Vetivert | Angelica seed<br>Cypress<br>Frankincense<br>Juniper berry | Galbanum<br>Violet leaf | Geranium<br>Jasmine<br>Lavender<br>Neroli<br>Palmarosa<br>Petitgrain<br>Rose<br>Ylang Ylang | Peppermint<br>Spearmint<br>Mint | Pine needles |

# Essential Oil Scent Profiles

| Essential Oil | Plant type | Scent Group Strength / Intensity | Scent profile | Compatible Essential Oils | | |
|---|---|---|---|---|---|---|
| | | | | Top notes (most volatile, uplifting) | Middle notes (body notes, balancing) | Base notes (tenacious, lingering, grounding) |
| Angelica root | Herb<br>Dried roots and rhizomes | Amber<br>Medium | Green, weedy, amber, terpenic, incense, ambrette, musk, celery, spicy, vegetable notes, with rich herbaceous-earthy body notes. | Bergamot<br>Sweet Fennel<br>Ginger<br>Grapefruit<br>Lemon<br>Lime<br>Mandarin<br>Orange<br>Clary Sage | Helichrysum (Immortelle)<br>Black Pepper | Cedarwood Atlas<br>Patchouli<br>Sandalwood<br>Vetivert |
| Angelica seed | Seeds | Terpenic<br>High | Angelica, fresh, terpenic, peppery, earthy, spicy, anisic, ambrette, woody, musk, soapy, powdery | | | |
| Basil | Herb<br>Flowering tops and leaves<br>Lamiaceae (Labiatae) | Anisic – (for example, relating to or resulting from Anise)<br>Medium | Fresh, sweet, herbaceous, aniseed-like, tarragon-like, slightly green with warm balsamic-woody undertone and lingering faint, sweet to non-distinctive dry-out notes | Bergamot<br>Citronella<br>Galbanum<br>Grapefruit<br>Lemon<br>Lemongrass<br>Lime<br>Niaouli<br>Orange bitter<br>Petitgrain | Geranium<br>Hyssop<br>Lavender<br>Marjoram<br>Melissa<br>Black Pepper<br>Peppermint<br>Rosemary<br>Clary Sage | Cinnamon leaf<br>Galbanum<br>Sandalwood<br>Violet leaf (absolute) |
| Benzoin | Deciduous tree<br>Resin<br>Styracaceae | Balsamic<br>Medium | Intensely rich, sweet-balsamic, vanilla-like, camphoraceous, medicinal | Bergamot<br>Caraway<br>Cardamom<br>Coriander<br>Eucalyptus<br>Galbanum<br>Grapefruit<br>Lemon<br>Lime<br>Mandarin<br>Nutmeg<br>Orange bitter<br>Petitgrain | Cypress<br>Juniper berry<br>Myrtle<br>Black Pepper<br>Peppermint | Cinnamon<br>Frankincense<br>Jasmine<br>Myrrh<br>Neroli (orange blossom)<br>Rose<br>Sandalwood<br>Ylang Ylang |

| Essential Oil | Plant type | Scent Group — Strength / Intensity | Scent profile | Compatible Essential Oils — Top notes (most volatile, uplifting) | Middle notes (body notes, balancing) | Base notes (tenacious, lingering, grounding) |
|---|---|---|---|---|---|---|
| Bergamot | Evergreen tree<br>Sour fruits<br>Rutaceae | Citrus<br>Medium | Citrus, fresh, lemony-orange, sweet-fruity, green, slightly spicy-balsamic undertones | Basil<br>Cardamom<br>Cajeput<br>Caraway<br>Citronella<br>Coriander<br>Fennel<br>Ginger<br>Grapefruit<br>Lemon<br>Lemongrass<br>Lime<br>Mandarin<br>May Chang<br>Niaouli<br>Nutmeg<br>Orange bitter<br>Palmarosa<br>Petitgrain<br>Clary Sage<br>Tea Tree<br>Thyme | Carrot seed<br>Cedarwood<br>Chamomile(s)<br>Chaste Tree<br>Cypress<br>Geranium<br>Helichrysum<br>Hyssop<br>Juniper berry<br>Lavender<br>Marjoram<br>Melissa<br>Myrtle<br>Oregano<br>Black Pepper<br>Peppermint<br>Rosemary<br>Turpentine<br>Yarrow | Benzoin<br>Cinnamon leaf<br>Clove bud<br>Frankincense<br>Jasmine<br>Myrrh<br>Neroli (orange blossom)<br>Patchouli<br>Rose<br>Sandalwood<br>Spikenard<br>Turmeric<br>Valerian<br>Vetivert<br>Violet (absolute)<br>Ylang Ylang |
| Cajeput | Evergreen tree<br>Fresh leaves and twigs<br>Myrtaceae | Herbal<br>Medium | Mild, sweet-fruity, fresh, rosemary, camphoraceous, menthol, metallic, with an herbaceous green, woody odour, then very faint herbaceous dry-out notes. | Bergamot<br>Eucalyptus<br>Grapefruit<br>Lemon<br>Lime<br>Mandarin<br>Niaouli<br>Orange bitter<br>Petitgrain<br>Tea Tree<br>Thyme | Cypress<br>Juniper berry<br>Lavender<br>Marjoram<br>Myrtle<br>Rosemary | Cedarwood Atlas<br>Rose<br><br>(see Myrtle and Tea Tree profiles below for further potential base notes) |

| Name | Plant / Part / Family | Note | Aroma | Blends with | | |
|---|---|---|---|---|---|---|
| Caraway | Aromatic annual herb; Ripe seeds or fruits (crushed); Apiaceae (Umbelliferae) | Herbal; Medium | Fresh, herbal, spicy, minty, balsamic, rye-bread, carvones, seedy, carroty. Very overpowering – use in moderation | Bergamot, Cardamom, Coriander, Fennel, Galbanum, Ginger, Grapefruit, Lemon, Lime, Mandarin, Nutmeg, Orange | Geranium, Black Pepper, Peppermint, Petitgrain | Cedarwood Atlas, Benzoin, Cassia, Cinnamon leaf, Clove bud, Frankincense, Jasmine, Neroli (orange blossom), Patchouli, Rose, Turmeric, Ylang Ylang |
| Cardamom | Perennial reed-like herb; Dried ripe fruits / seeds; Zingiberaceae | Spicy; Medium | Warm, camphoraceous, medicinal, eucalyptus, sweet and spicy, warming, with wood-balsamic undertones. | Bergamot, Caraway, Coriander, Fennel, Grapefruit, Ginger, Lemon, Lime, Mandarin, Nutmeg, Orange bitter, Peppermint, Petitgrain, Tea Tree, Thyme | Cypress, Geranium, Black Pepper, Rosemary, Clary Sage | Benzoin, Cedarwood Atlas, Cinnamon leaf, Clove bud, Frankincense, Jasmine, Neroli (orange blossom), Rose, Sandalwood, Spikenard, Turmeric, Ylang Ylang |
| Carrot Seed | Herbaceous plant; Dried fruits / seeds; Apiaceae (Umbelliferae) | Herbal; High | Dry, carrot-like, sweet, fresh, cumin, spicy, green, woody, earthy, fungal-like, slightly herbaceous to slightly peppery at dry-out. | Bergamot, Grapefruit, Lemon, Lime, Mandarin, Orange, Petitgrain | Geranium, Lavender, Black Pepper | Cedarwood Atlas, Cassie, Neroli (orange blossom), Patchouli, Rose, Sandalwood |

| Essential Oil | Plant type | Scent Group Strength / Intensity | Scent profile | Compatible Essential Oils | | |
| --- | --- | --- | --- | --- | --- | --- |
| | | | | Top notes (most volatile, uplifting) | Middle notes (body notes, balancing) | Base notes (tenacious, lingering, grounding) |
| Cedarwood Atlas | Cone-bearing evergreen tree<br><br>Wood, stumps and sawdust<br><br>Pinaceae | Woody<br><br>Medium | Dry, woody, herbaceous, with camphoraceous top notes and sweet, tenacious wood-balsamic undertones, with a mile wood dry-out scent. | Bergamot<br>Cajiput<br>Cardamom<br>Caraway<br>Citronella<br>Coriander<br>Eucalyptus<br>Ginger<br>Grapefruit<br>Lemongrass<br>Mandarin<br>May Chang<br>Niaouli<br>Orange bitter<br>Palmarosa<br>Petitgrain<br>Clary Sage | Carrot seed<br>Chamomile Roman<br>Cypress<br>Geranium<br>Helichrysum<br>Juniper berry<br>Lavender<br>Marjoram<br>Myrtle<br>Oregano<br>Pine<br>Rosemary<br>Turpentine<br>Yarrow | Cassie<br>Frankincense<br>Jasmine<br>Neroli (orange blossom)<br>Patchouli<br>Rose<br>Rosewood<br>Sandalwood<br>Valerian<br>Vetivert<br>Ylang Ylang<br><br>Other oriental and floral base notes |
| Chamomile German | Strongly aromatic annual plant / herb<br><br>Flowering heads<br><br>Asteraceae (Compositae) | Herbal<br><br>High | Herbaceous, sweet, medicinal, phenolic, fruity, green, warm, intense, hay-like, with warm, tobacco-like dry-out notes. | Bergamot<br>Grapefruit<br>Lemon<br>Lime<br>Mandarin<br>Orange bitter<br>Petitgrain<br>Clary Sage | Geranium<br>Lavender<br>Marjoram<br>Melissa<br>Yarrow | Myrrh<br>Neroli (orange blossom)<br>Patchouli<br>Rose<br>Turmeric<br>Valerian |
| Chamomile German | Aromatic perennial flowering plant / herb<br><br>Flowering heads<br><br>Asteraceae (Compositae) | Herbal<br><br>High | Sweet, fruity (like ripe apple), herbaceous, green, spicy, woody, and cognac-like, with warm, tea-like dry-out notes. | Bergamot<br>Grapefruit<br>Lavender<br>Lemon<br>Lime<br>Mandarin<br>Orange bitter<br>Petitgrain<br>Clary Sage | Cypress<br>Geranium<br>Helichrysum<br>Marjoram<br>Melissa<br>Yarrow | Cedarwood Atlas<br>Jasmine<br>Neroli (orange blossom)<br>Patchouli<br>Rose<br>Spikenard<br>Valarian |

| Name | Botanical description | Type | Note | Aroma | Blends with (citrus) | Blends with (herb/floral) | Blends with (other) |
|---|---|---|---|---|---|---|---|
| Chaste Tree Vitex Agnus Castus | Fragrant, deciduous shrub or tree / Fruits or leaves / Lamiaceae (formerly Verbenaceae) | Herbal | Medium | Cannabis-like and eucalyptus top notes, with floral, warm, fresh, peppery, sweet, spicy body notes and lemon-like, woody undertones and dry-out notes. | Bergamot, Grapefruit, Lemon, Lime, Mandarin, Orange | Geranium, Lavender, Black Pepper | Neroli (orange blossom), Rose, Ylang Ylang |
| Cinnamon Bark / Leaf | Tropical evergreen tree / Leaves and twigs / Lauraceae | Spicy | Medium | Woody, spicy, clove, cinnamon, with a warm but slightly harsh tone, and warm-spicy, clove-like dry-out notes. | Basil, Bergamot, Caraway, Cardamom, Coriander, Ginger, Grapefruit, Lemon, Lime, Mandarin, Nutmeg, Orange, Petitgrain, Tea Tree, Thyme | Geranium, Lavender, Black Pepper, Peppermint, Rosemary | Benzoin, Clove bud, Frankincense, Jasmine, Myrrh, Neroli (orange blossom), Rose, Spikenard, Turmeric, Ylang Ylang, Oriental type oils |
| Citronella | Tall, erect, aromatic perennial grass / Fresh or partially dried leaves / Poaceae (Gramineae) | Citrus | Medium | Fresh, sweet, geraniol, lemony, green, grassy-woody. | Basil, Bergamot, Grapefruit, Lemon, Lime, Mandarin, Niaouli, Orange bitter, Palmarosa, Thyme | Geranium, Lavender, Oregano, Black Pepper, Pine, Rosemary | Cedarwood Atlas, Rose, Sandalwood |

| Essential Oil | Plant type | Scent Group Strength / Intensity | Scent profile | Compatible Essential Oils | | |
|---|---|---|---|---|---|---|
| | | | | Top notes (most volatile, uplifting) | Middle notes (body notes, balancing) | Base notes (tenacious, lingering, grounding) |
| Clove Bud | Slender evergreen tree  Dried flower buds, leaves or stalks and stems  Myrtaceae | Spicy  Medium | Bud: fresh, fruity, top note, sweet, spicy, balsamic, woody, minty, phenolic, with warm spicy woody dry-out notes.  Leaf: spicy, aromatic, woody, balsamic, minty, peppery, phenolic, and powdery, with clove-like, dry-out notes.  Stalks and stems: spicy, aromatic, woody, minty, fatty, phenolic, and powdery, with clove-like dry-out notes. | Bergamot Caraway Cardamom Coriander Coumarin Ginger Grapefruit Lemon Lemongrass Lime Mandarin Nutmeg Orange bitter Palmarosa Petitgrain Tea Tree | Geranium Helichrysum Lavender Melissa Myrtle Black Pepper Peppermint Rosemary | Cinnamon leaf Myrrh Neroli (orange blossom) Patchouli Rose Sandalwood Turmeric Ylang Ylang |
| Coriander | Strongly aromatic herb  Ripe seeds (crushed)  Apiaceae (Umbelliferae) | Spicy  Medium | Seed: fresh, sweet, floral, herbal, rose-woody, woody-spicy, blueberry, green, terpenic.  Leaf: green, fatty, aldehydic, citrus-like, with brown (woody-nutty) herbal nuances. | *Seed:* Bergamot Caraway Cardamom Citronella Fennel Galbanum Grapefruit Ginger Lemon Lime Lemongrass Mandarin Nutmeg Niaouli Orange orang bitter Clary Sage Lemon-scented Tea Tree  *Leaf:* Basil Bergamot Lemon Tea Tree | *Seed:* Cypress Geranium Black Pepper Peppermint Petitgrain Pine  *Leaf:* Geranium Marjoram | *Seed:* Benzoin Cedarwood Atlas Cinnamon leaf Clove bud Frankincense Jasmine Neroli (orange blossom) Rose Sandalwood Spikenard  *Leaf:* Turmeric Ylang Ylang |

| | | | | | | |
|---|---|---|---|---|---|---|
| Cypress | Statuesque, cone-shaped tree<br>Twigs, needles, sometimes cones<br>Cupressaceae | Terpenic<br>Medium | Fresh, pine, woody, earthy, dry, spicy, cedar-like, and gently camphoraceous, with sweet, balsamic dry-out notes. | Bergamot<br>Cajeput<br>Cardamom<br>Coriander<br>Grapefruit<br>Lemon<br>Lime<br>Mandarin<br>Niaouli<br>Orange bitter<br>Petitgrain<br>Lemon-scented Tea Tree | Cedarwood<br>Chamomile (Maroc, Roman)<br>Geranium<br>Juniper berry<br>Lavender<br>Marjoram<br>Melissa<br>Black Pepper<br>Pine<br>Turpentine | Benzoin<br>Frankincense<br>Jasmine<br>Myrrh<br>Patchouli<br>Rose<br>Sandalwood<br>Spikenard |
| Eucalyptus | Diverse genus of flowering, tall, green trees and shrubs<br>Partially dried leaves and young twigs<br>Myrtaceae | Herbal<br>High | Herbal, eucalyptus, camphoraceous, medicinal, with a woody undertone. | Cajeput<br>Grapefruit<br>Lavender<br>Lemon<br>Lime<br>Niaouli<br>Orange bitter<br>Tea Tree<br>Thyme | Geranium<br>Marjoram<br>Myrtle<br>Peppermint<br>Pine<br>Rosemary<br>Turpentine<br>Yarrow | Cedarwood<br>Benzoin<br><br>*(see Myrtle and Tea Tree for further potential base notes)* |
| Fennel | Aromatic biennial or perennial herb<br>Sweet: Crushed seeds<br>Bitter: Crushed seeds, whole plant<br>Apiaceae (Umbelliferae) | Anisic – *(for example, relating to or resulting from Anise)*<br>Medium | Sweet Fennel: very sweet, earthy, anise-like, green, peppery, herbal, spicy, with warm, aniseed-like dry-out notes.<br>Bitter Fennel: sharp, warm, camphoraceous | Bergamot<br>Caraway<br>Cardamom<br>Coriander<br>Galbanum<br>Grapefruit<br>Lemon<br>Lime<br>Mandarin<br>Niaouli<br>Orange | Geranium<br>Lavender<br>Peppermint<br>Black Pepper | Neroli (orange blossom)<br>Rose<br>Sandalwood<br><br>*(see Galbanum's profile for further potential base notes)* |

| Essential Oil | Plant type | Scent Group Strength / Intensity | Scent profile | Compatible Essential Oils Top notes (most volatile, uplifting) | Middle notes (body notes, balancing) | Base notes (tenacious, lingering, grounding) |
|---|---|---|---|---|---|---|
| Frankincense | Small Tree with papery, peeling bark<br><br>Resin<br><br>Burseraceae | Terpenic<br><br>Medium | Fresh, terpenic, lemony, green, resinous, with persistent, balsamic-herbaceous dry-out notes | Basil<br>Bergamot<br>Caraway<br>Cardamom<br>Coriander<br>Galbanum<br>Ginger<br>Grapefruit<br>Lemon<br>Lime<br>Mandarin<br>May Chang<br>Orange bitter<br>Palmarosa<br>Petitgrain<br>Clary Sage | Cypress<br>Geranium<br>Helichrysum<br>Lavender<br>Melissa<br>Myrtle<br>Black Pepper<br>Pine<br>Rosemary<br>Turpentine | Benzoin<br>Cedarwood Atlas<br>Cinnamon leaf<br>Jasmine<br>Myrrh<br>Neroli (orange blossom)<br>Rose<br>Sandalwood<br>Spikenard<br>Turmeric<br>Vetivert<br>Ylang Ylang |
| Galbanum | Large perennial herb<br><br>Oleo gum resin<br><br>Apeaceae (Umbelliferae) | Green<br><br>High | Fresh, green, earthy, rooty, woody, balsamic, metallic, with balsamic agrestic to dry-earthy and spicy dry-out notes | Basil<br>Bergamot<br>Grapefruit<br>Lemon<br>Lime<br>Mandarin<br>Orange bitter<br>Petitgrain | Geranium<br>Lavender<br>Juniper Berry<br>Myrtle<br>Pine | Benzoin<br>Frankincense<br>Jasmine<br>Myrrh<br>Neroli (orange blossom)<br>Rose<br>Sandalwood<br>Ylang Ylang |

| | | | | | | |
|---|---|---|---|---|---|---|
| Geranium | Hairy perennial shrub (numerous species)<br>Leaves, stalks, flowers<br>Geraniaceae | Floral<br>Medium | Rich, floral, rose-like, sweet, and minty, with a hint of lemon and greens (green leaves, such as violet leaves or galbanum resin), finishing with green and rose-like dry-out notes. | Basil<br>Bergamot<br>Caraway<br>Cardamom<br>Citronella<br>Coriander<br>Eucalyptus<br>Fennel<br>Galbanum<br>Ginger<br>Grapefruit<br>Lemon<br>Lemongrass<br>Lime<br>Mandarin<br>May Chang<br>Niaouli<br>Nutmeg<br>Orange bitter<br>Palmarosa<br>Petitgrain<br>Clary Sage<br>Tea Tree | Carrot seed<br>Chaste Tree<br>Chamomile(s)<br>Cypress<br>Helichrysum<br>Hyssop<br>Juniper berry<br>Lavender<br>Marjoram<br>Melissa<br>Oregano<br>Myrtle<br>Black Pepper<br>Peppermint<br>Yarrow | Cinnamon leaf<br>Cedarwood Atlas<br>Clove bud<br>Frankincense<br>Jasmine<br>Myrrh<br>Neroli (orange blossom)<br>Patchouli<br>Rose<br>Sandalwood<br>Spikenard<br>Turmeric<br>Valerian<br>Vetivert |
| Ginger | Reed-like perennial<br>Unpeeled, dried and ground roots<br>Zingiberaceae | Spicy<br>Medium | Fresh, slightly green, spicy-woody, terpenic, warm, citrusy, and mellow, with coriander-like tones and warm, balsamic, floral-woody dry-out notes. | Bergamot<br>Caraway<br>Cardamom<br>Coriander<br>Grapefruit<br>Lemon<br>Lemongrass<br>Lime<br>Mandarin<br>May Chang<br>Nutmeg<br>Orange bitter<br>Palmarosa<br>Petitgrain | Geranium<br>Marjoram<br>Melissa<br>Myrtle<br>Black Pepper<br>Peppermint<br>Rosemary | Cedarwood Atlas<br>Cinnamon leaf<br>Clove bud<br>Frankincense<br>Jasmine<br>Myrrh<br>Neroli (orange blossom)<br>Patchouli<br>Rose<br>Rosewood<br>Sandalwood<br>Turmeric<br>Vetivert<br>Ylang Ylang |

| Essential Oil | Plant type | Scent Group Strength / Intensity | Scent profile | Compatible Essential Oils | | |
|---|---|---|---|---|---|---|
| | | | | Top notes (most volatile, uplifting) | Middle notes (body notes, balancing) | Base notes (tenacious, lingering, grounding) |
| Grapefruit | Evergreen tree<br><br>Fresh fruit peel<br><br>Rutaceae | Citrus<br><br>Medium | Fresh, sweet, dry, citrus, with faint, nondescript dry-out notes | Basil<br>Bergamot<br>Cajeput<br>Caraway<br>Cardamom<br>Citronella<br>Coriander<br>Eucalyptus<br>Fennel<br>Galbanum<br>Ginger<br>Lemon<br>Lemongrass<br>Lime<br>Mandarin<br>May Chang<br>Niaouli<br>Nutmeg<br>Orange bitter<br>Palmarosa<br>Petitgrain<br>Clary Sage<br>Lemon-scented Tea Tree<br>Thyme | Carrot seed<br>Chamomile(s)<br>Chaste Tree<br>Cypress<br>Geranium<br>Helichrysum<br>Juniper berry<br>Lavender<br>Marjoram<br>Melissa<br>Myrtle<br>Oregano<br>Black Pepper<br>Peppermint<br>Pine<br>Rosemary<br>Turpentine | Benzoin<br>Cedarwood Atlas<br>Cinnamon leaf<br>Clove bud<br>Frankincense<br>Jasmine<br>Myrrh<br>Neroli (orange blossom)<br>Patchouli<br>Rose<br>Sandalwood<br>Spikenard<br>Turmeric<br>Valerian<br>Vetivert<br>Yarrow<br>Ylang Ylang |
| Helichrysum (Immortelle) | Strongly aromatic herb<br><br>Fresh flowers and flowering tops<br><br>Asteraceae (Compositae) | Herbal<br><br>Medium | Sweet, fruity, honey-like, warm, herbal, woody, floral, coumarinic, with delicate, tea-like undertones and dry-out notes | Bergamot<br>Coumarin<br>Grapefruit<br>Lemon<br>Lime<br>Mandarin<br>Orange<br>Petitgrain<br>Clary Sage | Chamomile(s)<br>Geranium<br>Juniper berry<br>Lavender<br>Melissa<br>Yarrow | Cedarwood<br>Clove bud<br>Frankincense<br>Neroli (orange blossom)<br>Peru Balsam<br>Rose<br>Turmeric<br>Ylang Ylang |

| | | | | | | |
|---|---|---|---|---|---|---|
| Hyssop | Small, semi-evergreen, perennial shrub or subshrub<br><br>Fresh leaves and flowering tops<br><br>Lamiaceae (Labiatae) | Herbal<br><br>Medium | Herbal, like sage and clary sage, camphoraceous, green, piney, terpenic, woody, with warm, spicy-herbaceous body notes and fading undertones and dry-out notes | Basil<br>Bergamot<br>Grapefruit<br>Lemon<br>Lime<br>Mandarin<br>Orange<br>Clary Sage | Geranium<br>Lavender<br>Melissa<br>Myrtle<br>Rosemary | Neroli (orange blossom)<br><br>*(see Clary Sage's profile for further potential base notes)* |
| Jasmine | Either deciduous or evergreen climbing shrubs<br><br>Fresh flowers<br><br>Oleaceae | Floral<br><br>Medium | Intensely rich, yet delicate, ethereal, sweet, warm, balsamic, fruity, and green, with tenacious, floral, tea-like undertones and dry-out notes<br><br>Rounds out any rough or sharp notes and aromatically blends with most other oils | Bergamot<br>Cardamom<br>Caraway<br>Coriander<br>Galbanum<br>Ginger<br>Grapefruit<br>Lemon<br>Lime<br>Lemongrass<br>Mandarin<br>May Chang<br>Nutmeg<br>Orange, bitter<br>Palmarosa<br>Petitgrain<br>Clary Sage | Chamomile Roman<br>Cypress<br>Geranium<br>Lavender<br>Marjoram<br>Melissa<br>Myrtle<br>Oregano<br>Black Pepper | Benzoin<br>Cinnamon leaf<br>Frankincense<br>Myrrh<br>Neroli (orange blossom)<br>Patchouli<br>Rose<br>Sandalwood<br>Turmeric<br>Vetivert<br>Ylang Ylang |
| Juniper Berry | Coniferous evergreen shrub that differs in shape and size depending on its environment<br><br>Berries<br>Needles and wood<br><br>Cupressaceae | Terpenic<br><br>Medium | Fresh, balsamic, terpenic, warm and woody, carrot-seedy and peppery, with sweet, warm, balsamic dry-out notes | Benzoin<br>Bergamot<br>Cajeput<br>Galbanum<br>Geranium<br>Grapefruit<br>Lemon<br>Lime<br>Mandarin<br>Niaouli<br>Orange bitter<br>Clary Sage | Cypress<br>Helichrysum<br>Lavender<br>Pine<br>Rosemary<br>Yarrow | Cedarwood Atlas<br>Myrrh<br>Sandalwood<br>Vetivert<br><br>*(see also Cedarwood and Cypress's profile for further potential base and middle notes)* |

| Essential Oil | Plant type | Scent Group Strength / Intensity | Scent profile | Compatible Essential Oils | | |
|---|---|---|---|---|---|---|
| | | | | Top notes (most volatile, uplifting) | Middle notes (body notes, balancing) | Base notes (tenacious, lingering, grounding) |
| Lavender | Small, woody, evergreen shrub<br><br>Fresh flowering tops<br><br>Lamiaceae (Labiatae) | Angustifolia / Spike: Floral<br><br>Medium | Angustifolia: fresh, floral, fruity to herbaceous, spicy, camphoraceous, aldehydic, and balsamic-woody undertones to nondescript dry-out notes<br><br>English lavender angustifolia softer, mellower, slightly rounder notes compared to French lavenders and other lavender oils<br><br>Spike: fresh and strongly camphoraceous, with herbaceous-woody dry-out notes (sometimes described as a cross between sage and lavender) | Basil<br>Bergamot<br>Cajeput<br>Chaste Tree<br>Citronella<br>Cypress<br>Eucalyptus<br>Fennel<br>Galbanum<br>Grapefruit<br>Lemon<br>Lemongrass<br>Lime<br>Mandarin<br>May Chang<br>Niaouli<br>Orange bitter<br>Palmarosa<br>Petitgrain<br>Clary Sage<br>Tea Tree<br>Thyme | Carrot seed<br>Cedarwood<br>Chamomile(s)<br>Geranium<br>Helichrysum<br>Hyssop<br>Juniper berry<br>Marjoram<br>Melissa<br>Myrtle<br>Oregano<br>Peppermint<br>Pine<br>Black Pepper<br>Rosemary<br>Turpentine<br>Yarrow | Cinnamon leaf<br>Clove bud<br>Frankincense<br>Jasmine<br>May Chang<br>Neroli (orange blossom)<br>Myrrh<br>Patchouli<br>Rose<br>Sandalwood<br>Spikenard<br>Turmeric<br>Valarian<br>Vetivert<br>Ylang Ylang |

| Name | Description | Category | Note | Scent | Blends with | | |
|---|---|---|---|---|---|---|---|
| Lemon | Small evergreen tree or spreading shrub; Outer peel of the fresh fruit; Rutaceae | Citrus | Medium | Light, fresh, citrus scent, reminiscent of lemon peel | Basil, Bergamot, Cajeput, Caraway, Cardamom, Citronella, Coriander, Eucalyptus, Fennel, Galbanum, Grapefruit, Ginger, Lime, Lemongrass, Mandarin, May Chang, Niaouli, Nutmeg, Orange bitter, Palmarosa, Petitgrain, Clary Sage, Lemon-scented Tea Tree, Thyme | Carrot seed, Chamomile(s), Chaste Tree, Cypress, Geranium, Helichrysum, Hyssop, Juniper berry, Lavender, Melissa, Myrtle, Oregano, Black Pepper, Peppermint, Pine, Rosemary, Turpentine, Yarrow | Benzoin, Cinnamon leaf, Clove bud, Frankincense, Jasmine, Myrrh, Neroli (orange blossom), Patchouli, Rose, Sandalwood, Spikenard, Turmeric, Valerian, Vetivert, Ylang Ylang |
| Lemongrass | An aromatic, sweet, lemon-scented perennial grass; Fresh or partially dried, finely chopped leaves or grass; Poaceae (Gramineae) | Citrus | Medium | Fresh, sweet, lemony, grassy, rosy, tomato leaf, with earthy undertones, with lemony, herbal, green tea-like body notes and herbaceous, oily, dry-out notes | Basil, Bergamot, Coriander, Ginger, Grapefruit, Lemon, Lime, Mandarin, May Chang, Nutmeg, Orange bitter, Palmarosa, Petitgrain, Tea Tree, Thyme | Geranium, Lavender, Marjoram, Melissa, Myrtle, Niaouli, Oregano, Black Pepper, Peppermint, Pine, Rosemary | Cedarwood Atlas, Jasmine, Neroli (orange blossom), Patchouli, Rose, Sandalwood, Turmeric, Vetivert, Ylang Ylang |

## Compatible Essential Oils

| Essential Oil | Plant type | Scent Group Strength / Intensity | Scent profile | Top notes (most volatile, uplifting) | Middle notes (body notes, balancing) | Base notes (tenacious, lingering, grounding) |
|---|---|---|---|---|---|---|
| Mandarin | A small evergreen, usually thorny tree<br><br>Outer peel of the fresh fruit<br><br>Rutaceae | Citrus<br><br>Medium | Citrus, floral, terpenic, aldehyde, intensely fruity, sweet, fresh, deep, softly citrussy with obvious mandarin peel odour fading to a faintly fruity, tangeriney, soft and round, herbaceous-fruity scent, until barely detectable | Bergamot<br>Cajeput<br>Caraway<br>Cardamom<br>Citronella<br>Coriander<br>Fennel<br>Ginger<br>Galbanum<br>Grapefruit<br>Lemon<br>Lemongrass<br>Lime<br>May Chang<br>Niaouli<br>Nutmeg<br>Orange bitter<br>Palmarosa<br>Petitgrain<br>Clary Sage<br>Tea Tree<br>Thyme | Carrot seed<br>Cedarwood<br>Chamomile(s)<br>Chaste Tree<br>Cypress<br>Geranium<br>Helichrysum<br>Hyssop<br>Juniper berry<br>Lavender<br>Marjoram<br>Melissa<br>Myrtle<br>Oregano<br>Black Pepper<br>Peppermint<br>Pine<br>Rosemary<br>Yarrow | Benzoin<br>Cinnamon leaf<br>Clove bud<br>Frankincense<br>Jasmine<br>Neroli (orange blossom)<br>Myrrh<br>Patchouli<br>Rose<br>Sandalwood<br>Spikenard<br>Turmeric<br>Valerian<br>Vetivert<br>Ylang Ylang |
| Marjoram | A bushy, herbaceous plant<br><br>Flowering leaves and tops<br><br>Lamiaceae (Labiate) | Spicy<br><br>Medium | Spicy, fresh, green, herbal, minty, camphoraceous, then warm and woody, with camphoraceous-spicy dry-out notes | Basil<br>Bergamot<br>Cajeput<br>Eucalyptus<br>Ginger<br>Grapefruit<br>Lemongrass<br>Mandarin<br>Niaouli<br>Orange bitter<br>Petitgrain<br>Clary Sage<br>Tea Tree<br>Thyme | Chamomile(s)<br>Cypress<br>Geranium<br>Lavender<br>Melissa<br>Oregano<br>Black Pepper<br>Peppermint<br>Pine<br>Rosemary | Cedarwood Atlas<br>Jasmine<br>Myrrh<br>Neroli (orange blossom)<br>Rose<br>Sandalwood<br>Vetivert<br>Ylang Ylang |

| Oil | Description | Note | Aroma | Blends well with | | |
|---|---|---|---|---|---|---|
| May Chang | A small evergreen tropical tree or shrub<br>Leaves<br>Lauraceae | Citrus<br>Medium | Intense, lemony, green, lemongrass-like, aldehydic, with sweet, fresh undertones and sharp, lemony dry-out notes. | Bergamot<br>Ginger<br>Grapefruit<br>Lemon<br>Lemongrass<br>Lime<br>Mandarin<br>Nutmeg<br>Niaouli<br>Orange bitter<br>Palmarosa<br>Petitgrain<br>Tea tree<br>Thyme | Geranium<br>Juniper berry<br>Lavender<br>Black Pepper<br>Rosemary | Cedarwood Atlas<br>Frankincense<br>Jasmine<br>Neroli (orange blossom)<br>Patchouli<br>Rose<br>Sandalwood<br>Vetivert<br>Ylang Ylang |
| Melissa (Lemon Balm) | A sweet lemon-scented herb related to mint<br>Leaves and flowering tops<br>Lamiaceae (Labiatae) | Citrus<br>Medium | Sweet, citrus, citronella, herby, grassy, with fresh, lemony notes and weak citrussy dry-out notes | Basil<br>Bergamot<br>Ginger<br>Grapefruit<br>Lemon<br>Lemongrass (*substitute*)<br>Lime<br>Mandarin<br>Niaouli<br>Nutmeg<br>Orange bitter<br>Petitgrain<br>Thyme | Chamomile(s)<br>Cypress<br>Geranium<br>Helichrysum<br>Hyssop<br>Lavender<br>Marjoram<br>Myrtle<br>Black Pepper<br>Peppermint<br>Pine<br>Rosemary | Clove bud<br>Frankincense<br>Jasmine<br>Myrrh<br>Neroli (orange blossom)<br>Patchouli<br>Rose<br>Sandalwood<br>Vetivert<br>Ylang Ylang |
| Myrrh | A small, thorny deciduous shrub<br>Resin<br>Burseraceae | Balsamic<br>Medium | Distilled: balsamic, dry, toffee, metallic, slightly medicated, resinous, mushroomy, with warm-spicy body notes and nondescript dry-out notes<br><br>Absolute: warm, rich, spicy, balsamic tones, with lingering warm, spicy, balsamic dry-out notes | Bergamot<br>Galbanum<br>Ginger<br>Grapefruit<br>Lemon<br>Lime<br>Mandarin<br>Nutmeg<br>Orange bitter<br>Palmarosa<br>Petitgrain<br>Clary Sage<br>Tea Tree | Chamomile German<br>Cypress<br>Geranium<br>Juniper berry<br>Lavender<br>Marjoram<br>Melissa<br>Myrtle<br>Peppermint<br>Pine<br>Rosemary<br>Thyme | Benzoin<br>Cinnamon leaf<br>Clove bud<br>Frankincense<br>Jasmine<br>Neroli (orange blossom)<br>Patchouli<br>Rose<br>Sandalwood<br>Spikenard<br>Turmeric<br>Ylang Ylang |

| Essential Oil | Plant type | Scent Group Strength / Intensity | Scent profile | Compatible Essential Oils | | |
|---|---|---|---|---|---|---|
| | | | | Top notes (most volatile, uplifting) | Middle notes (body notes, balancing) | Base notes (tenacious, lingering, grounding) |
| Myrtle | A bushy, medium-sized evergreen shrub or small tree<br><br>Leaves, twigs, and sometimes flowers<br><br>Myrtaceae | Herbal<br><br>Medium | Fresh–camphoraceous, fruity, spicy, sweet, herbaceous; similar to eucalyptus, with warm camphoraceous body tones and faint, herbaceous, non-descript dry-out notes | Bergamot<br>Cajeput<br>Coriander<br>Eucalyptus<br>Galbanum<br>Ginger<br>Grapefruit<br>Lemon<br>Lime<br>Mandarin<br>Nutmeg<br>Orange bitter<br>Tea Tree | Geranium<br>Hyssop<br>Jasmine<br>Lavender<br>Melissa<br>Niaouli<br>Black Pepper<br>Rosemary<br>Clary Sage | Benzoin<br>Cedarwood Atlas<br>Clove bud<br>Frankincense<br>Myrrh<br>Neroli (orange blossom)<br>Rose<br>Ylang Ylang |
| Neroli | An evergreen fruit bearing tree<br><br>Freshly picked blossoms<br><br>Rutaceae | Floral<br><br>Medium | Distilled: sweet, characteristically reminiscent of orange flowers, citrussy, mandarin-like, petitgrain, herbal, with light, floral herbaceous, slightly citrussy middle tones (notes) and faint, non-descript dry-out notes<br><br>Absolute: fresh, delicate but rich, warm, with lingering, warm, floral-citrus dry-out notes | Distilled:<br>Bergamot<br>Caraway<br>Cardamom<br>Coriander<br>Fennel<br>Galbanum<br>Ginger<br>Grapefruit<br>Lemon<br>Lemongrass<br>Lime<br>Mandarin<br>May Chang<br>Niaouli<br>Orange bitter<br>Petitgrain<br>Clary Sage<br><br>Absolute:<br>All citrus oils | Distilled:<br>Carrot seed<br>Chamomile(s)<br>Chaste Tree<br>Geranium<br>Helichrysum<br>Hyssop<br>Lavender<br>Marjoram<br>Melissa<br>Myrtle<br>Oregano<br>Black Pepper<br>Yarrow | Distilled:<br>Benzoin<br>Cedarwood Atlas<br>Cinnamon leaf<br>Clove bud<br>Frankincense<br>Jasmine<br>Myrrh<br>Patchouli<br>Rose<br>Sandalwood<br>Spikenard<br>Turmeric<br>Vetivert<br>Ylang Ylang<br><br>Absolute:<br>Benzoin<br>Jasmine<br>Myrrh |

| | | | | | | |
|---|---|---|---|---|---|---|
| Niaouli | A medium-sized evergreen tree with a papery bark<br><br>Leaves and young twigs<br><br>Myrtaceae | Herbal<br><br>Medium | Sweet, camphoraceous, eucalyptus, minty, woody resinous | Cajeput<br>Citronella<br>Eucalyptus<br>Fennel<br>Grapefruit<br>Lemon<br>Lemongrass<br>Lime<br>Mandarin<br>May Chang<br>Orange bitter<br>Petitgrain<br>Tea Tree<br>Thyme | Cypress<br>Geranium<br>Juniper berry<br>Lavender<br>Marjoram<br>Melissa<br>Myrtle<br>Peppermint<br>Pine<br>Rosemary | Cedarwood Atlas<br><br>*(see Myrtle and Tea Tree's profile for further potential base notes)* |
| Nutmeg | A tropical evergreen tree<br><br>Dried seeds<br><br>An essential oil is also produced from the aril, or mace<br><br>Myristicaceae | Spicy<br><br>Medium | Sweet, warm, spicy, woody, characteristically nutmeg, powdery, pine, old wood, resinous, with terpenic top notes and warm, spicy-woody dry-out notes | Bergamot<br>Caraway<br>Cardamom<br>Coriander<br>Ginger<br>Grapefruit<br>Lemon<br>Lemongrass<br>Lime<br>Mandarin<br>May Chang<br>Orange bitter<br>Petitgrain<br>Tea Tree<br>Thyme | Geranium<br>Melissa<br>Black Pepper<br>Peppermint<br>Rosemary<br>Clary Sage | Benzoin<br>Cinnamon leaf<br>Clove bud<br>Jasmine<br>Myrrh<br>Patchouli<br>Rose<br>Spikenard<br>Turmeric |

| Essential Oil | Plant type | Scent Group / Strength / Intensity | Scent profile | Compatible Essential Oils | | |
|---|---|---|---|---|---|---|
| | | | | Top notes (most volatile, uplifting) | Middle notes (body notes, balancing) | Base notes (tenacious, lingering, grounding) |
| Orange bitter | Evergreen fruit bearing tree<br><br>Fruit peel from almost-ripe fruits<br><br>Rutaceae | Citrus<br><br>Medium | Fresh, orange-like, dry, woody, leafy, with slightly floral undertones and warm, non-descript dry-out notes | Bergamot<br>Basil<br>Caraway<br>Cardamon<br>Citronella<br>Coriander<br>Fennel<br>Galbanum<br>Ginger<br>Grapefruit<br>Lemon<br>Lemongrass<br>Lime<br>Mandarin<br>May Chang<br>Nutmeg<br>Palmarosa<br>Petitgrain<br>Clary Sage<br>Tea Tree<br>Thyme | Carrot Seed<br>Chamomile(s)<br>Chaste Tree<br>Cypress<br>Geranium<br>Helichrysum<br>Hyssop<br>Juniper berry<br>Lavender<br>Marjoram<br>Melissa<br>Myrtle<br>Niaouli<br>Oregano<br>Patchouli<br>Black Pepper<br>Peppermint<br>Pine<br>Rosemary<br>Yarrow | Benzoin<br>Cedarwood Atlas<br>Cinnamon leaf<br>Clove bud<br>Frankincense<br>Jasmine<br>Myrrh<br>Neroli (orange blossom)<br>Rose<br>Sandalwood<br>Spikenard<br>Turmeric<br>Valerian<br>Vetivert<br>Ylang Ylang |
| Oregano | A hardy perennial shrub-like herb with multiple branched stems (grows upright or as a creeping spread)<br><br>Dried leaves or dried leaves and flowering tops<br><br>Labiatae | Herbal<br><br>High | Thyme-like, green, herbaceous, warm, spicy, camphor, phenolic, and woody with warm, spicy, camphoraceous, woody middle notes and warm, spicy, woody dry-out notes | Bergamot<br>Citronella<br>Grapefruit<br>Lemon<br>Mandarin<br>Orange bitter<br>Petitgrain<br>Tea Tree<br>Thyme | Cypress<br>Geranium<br>Lavender (Spike)<br>Lemongrass<br>Marjoram<br>Melissa (lemon balm)<br>Peppermint<br>Pine<br>Rosemary | Cedarwood<br>Jasmine<br>Neroli<br>Rose<br>Sandalwood<br>Ylang Ylang |

| Name | Botanical | Note | Intensity | Aroma | Blends with | | |
|---|---|---|---|---|---|---|---|
| Palmarosa | A tall, herbaceous, fragrant (rose-like) tropical grass / Dried grass stems and leaves / Poaceae (Gramineae) | Floral | Medium | Sweet, floral, rosy, citrus, grassy, citronella, tomato, leafy, herbaceous, with rose / geranium-like undertones and faded, citrusy, non-descript dry-out notes | Bergamot, Citronella, Ginger, Grapefruit, Lemon, Lemongrass, Lime, Mandarin, May Chang, Niaouli, Orange bitter, Petitgrain, Tea Tree | Geranium, Lavender, Black Pepper | Cedarwood Atlas, Clove bud, Frankincense, Jasmine, Myrrh, Neroli (orange blossom), Patchouli, Rose, Sandalwood, Turmeric, Vetivert, Ylang Ylang |
| Patchouli | Perennial, fragrant, shrubby herb / Young, fresh, dried and partially fermented leaves / Lamiaceae (Labiatae) | Woody | Medium | Rich, sweet, herbaceous, mossy-woody, earthy, weedy, balsamic, spicy, minty to slightly camphoraceous-spicy, dry-woody, tenacious, with lingering dry-out notes | Bergamot, Ginger, Grapefruit, Lemongrass, Mandarin, Lemon, Lime, May Chang, Niaouli, Nutmeg, Orange bitter, Palmarosa, Petitgrain, Clary sage | Carrot seed, Chamomile(s), Cypress, Geranium, Lavender, Melissa | Clove bud, Cedarwood Atlas, Jasmine, Myrrh, Neroli (orange blossom), Rose, Sandalwood, Spikenard, Turmeric, Valerian, Vetivert, Ylang Ylang |

| Essential Oil | Plant type | Scent Group Strength / Intensity | Scent profile | Compatible Essential Oils | | |
|---|---|---|---|---|---|---|
| | | | | Top notes (most volatile, uplifting) | Middle notes (body notes, balancing) | Base notes (tenacious, lingering, grounding) |
| Black Pepper | A perennial woody climber or flowering vine<br><br>Dried, crushed peppercorns<br><br>Piperaceae | Spicy<br><br>Medium | Fresh, warm, spicy, terpenic, peppery, woody, with herbaceous undertones and mellow-peppery dry-out notes | Basil<br>Bergamot<br>Caraway<br>Cardamom<br>Citronella<br>Coriander<br>Fennel<br>Ginger<br>Grapefruit<br>Lemon<br>Lemongrass<br>Lime<br>Mandarin<br>May Chang<br>Nutmeg<br>Orange bitter<br>Palmarosa<br>Petitgrain<br>Clary Sage | Carrot seed<br>Chaste Tree<br>Cypress<br>Geranium<br>Lavender<br>Marjoram<br>Melissa<br>Rosemary<br>Yarrow | Cinnamon leaf<br>Clove bud<br>Benzoin<br>Frankincense<br>Jasmine<br>Neroli (orange blossom)<br>Rose<br>Sandalwood<br>Spikenard<br>Turmeric<br>Ylang Ylang |
| Peppermint | A seedless, or sterile, herbaceous hybrid plant (propagated via its roots)<br><br>Fresh leaves and flowers<br><br>Lamiaceae (Labiatae) | Minty<br><br>Medium | Cool, penetrating, pungent, pepper-minty, grassy-minty, with a grassy-minty-balsamic undertone and dry-herbaceous dry-out notes | Basil<br>Bergamot<br>Caraway<br>Cardamom<br>Coriander<br>Eucalyptus<br>Fennel<br>Grapefruit<br>Ginger<br>Lemon<br>Lemongrass<br>Lime<br>Mandarin<br>Niaouli<br>Nutmeg<br>Orange bitter<br>Petitgrain<br>Tea Tree<br>Yarrow | Geranium<br>Lavender<br>Marjoram<br>Melissa<br>Oregano<br>Pine<br>Rosemary | Benzoin<br>Cinnamon leaf<br>Clove<br>Myrrh<br>Rose<br>Sandalwood<br>Vetivert |

| Petitgrain | An evergreen, aromatic tree<br>Leaves and twigs<br>Rutacea | Floral<br>Medium | Floral, sage, neroli, citrus, sweet, fresh, woody-orange, green-mossy, with dry-herbaceous dry-out notes | Basil<br>Bergamot<br>Caraway<br>Cardamom<br>Cajeput<br>Coriander<br>Ginger<br>Grapefruit<br>Lemon<br>Lemongrass<br>Lime<br>Mandarin<br>May Chang<br>Niaouli<br>Nutmeg<br>Orange Bitter<br>Palmarosa<br>Tea Tree<br>Thyme | Carrot seed<br>Chamomile(s)<br>Cypress<br>Geranium<br>Helichrysum<br>Lavender<br>Marjoram<br>Melissa<br>Oregano<br>Peppermint<br>Black Pepper<br>Pine<br>Rosemary<br>Yarrow | Benzoin<br>Cedarwood Atlas<br>Cinnamon leaf<br>Clove bud<br>Frankincense<br>Jasmine<br>Myrrh<br>Neroli (orange blossom)<br>Patchouli<br>Rose<br>Sandalwood<br>Spikenard<br>Turmeric<br>Valerian<br>Ylang Ylang |
|---|---|---|---|---|---|---|
| Pine | A tall, evergreen, coniferous tree<br>Dried needles<br>Pinaceae | Earthy<br>Medium | Earthy, dry, weedy, pine-like, woody, resinous, with turpentine-like tones, balsamic body notes and non-descript at dry out. | Bergamot<br>Cajeput<br>Citronella<br>Coriander<br>Eucalyptus<br>Galbanum<br>Grapefruit<br>Lemon<br>Lime<br>Lemongrass<br>Mandarin<br>Orange bitter<br>Petitgrain<br>Clary Sage<br>Tea Tree<br>Thyme | Cypress<br>Juniper berry<br>Marjoram<br>Melissa<br>Oregano<br>Peppermint<br>Rosemary<br>Yarrow | Cedarwood Atlas<br>Frankincense<br>Myrrh<br>Sandalwood<br>Spikenard<br>Valerian |

| Essential Oil | Plant type | Scent Group Strength / Intensity | Scent profile | Compatible Essential Oils | | |
|---|---|---|---|---|---|---|
| | | | | Top notes (most volatile, uplifting) | Middle notes (body notes, balancing) | Base notes (tenacious, lingering, grounding) |
| Rosemary | An evergreen perennial bushy herb or shrub<br><br>Fresh flowering tops or whole plant<br><br>Lamiaceae (Labiatae) | Herbal<br><br>Medium | Strong, fresh, herbal, camphoraceous, woody, minty, balsamic, medicinal, phenolic, with woody-balsamic undertones and dry-herbaceous dry-out notes<br><br>Oxidized or poor-quality essential oils have a strong camphoraceous scent<br><br>*phenolic scent profile – Scent group: phenolic. Odour: plastic, rubbery | Bergamot<br>Basil<br>Cajeput<br>Cardamom<br>Citronella<br>Eucalyptus<br>Ginger<br>Grapefruit<br>Lemon<br>Lemongrass<br>Lime<br>Mandarin<br>May Chang<br>Niaouli<br>Nutmeg<br>Orange<br>Petitgrain bitter<br>Clary Sage<br>Tea Tree<br>Thyme | Hyssop<br>Juniper berry<br>Lavender<br>Marjoram<br>Melissa<br>Myrrh<br>Myrtle<br>Oregano<br>Black Pepper<br>Peppermint<br>Pine<br>Turpentine<br>Yarrow | Cedarwood Atlas<br>Cinnamon leaf<br>Clove bud<br>Frankincense<br>Rose<br>Valerian |
| Rose | A deciduous, informally shaped shrub<br><br>Fresh petals<br><br>Rosaceae | Floral<br><br>Medium | Intense, sweet, floral, rose, waxy, honey, spicy, green, *cortex, geranium, metallic, with rich, spicy, sweet, floral body notes and warm, floral, honey-like dry-out notes.<br><br>*cortex: green, earthy, leafy, nasturtium | Bergamot<br>Caraway<br>Cardamom<br>Cajeput<br>Citronella<br>Coriander<br>Fennel<br>Galbanum<br>Ginger<br>Grapefruit<br>Lemon<br>Lemongrass<br>Lime<br>Mandarin<br>Nutmeg<br>Orange bitter<br>Palmarosa<br>Petitgrain<br>Clary Sage<br>Tea Tree<br>Thyme | Carrot Seed<br>Chamomile(s)<br>Chaste Tree<br>Geranium<br>Helichrysum<br>Lavender<br>Marjoram<br>May Chang<br>Melissa<br>Myrtle<br>Oregano<br>Peppermint<br>Black Pepper<br>Rosemary<br>Yarrow | Benzoin<br>Cedarwood Atlas<br>Cinnamon leaf<br>Clove bud<br>Cypress<br>Frankincense<br>Jasmine<br>Myrrh<br>Neroli (orange blossom)<br>Patchouli<br>Sandalwood<br>Spikenard<br>Turmeric<br>Valarian<br>Vetivert<br>Ylang Ylang |

| | | | | | | |
|---|---|---|---|---|---|---|
| **Clary Sage** | A biennial or short-lived perennial herb, shrub, or subshrub<br><br>Flowering tops and leaves<br><br>Lamiaceae (Labiate) | Herbal<br><br>Medium | Fresh, herbal, tea, green, woody, weedy, dry, spicy, sage, powdery, with resinous-balsamic, herbaceous-woody body notes and dry-herbaceous dry-out notes | Basil<br>Bergamot<br>Cardamom<br>Coriander<br>Grapefruit<br>Lemon<br>Lime<br>Mandarin<br>Nutmeg<br>Orange bitter<br>Tea Tree<br>Thyme | Chamomile German<br>Geranium<br>Helichrysum<br>Hyssop<br>Juniper berry<br>Lavender<br>Marjoram<br>Myrtle<br>Black Pepper<br>Pine<br>Rosemary | Cedarwood Atlas<br>Frankincense<br>Jasmine<br>Myrrh<br>Neroli (orange blossom)<br>Patchouli<br>Rose<br>Sandalwood<br>Turmeric<br>Valerian<br>Vetivert<br>Ylang Ylang |
| **Sandalwood** | A semi-parasitic, slow growing tree<br><br>Pulverized heart wood, or milled sawdust<br><br>Santalaceae | Woody<br><br>Medium | Dry, woody, balsamic, sweet, myrrh, creamy, with non-descript top notes and soft, sweet, woody, balsamic, fatty-floral, very tenacious middle notes and faint dry-out notes | Basil<br>Bergamot<br>Cardamom<br>Citronella<br>Coriander<br>Fennel<br>Galbanum<br>Ginger<br>Grapefruit<br>Lemon<br>Lemongrass<br>Lime<br>Mandarin<br>May Chang<br>Orange bitter<br>Palmarosa<br>Petitgrain<br>Clary Sage | Carrot seed<br>Cypress<br>Geranium<br>Juniper berry<br>Lavender<br>Marjoram<br>Oregano<br>Black Pepper<br>Peppermint<br>Pine | Benzoin<br>Cedarwood Atlas<br>Clove bud<br>Frankincense<br>Jasmine<br>Myrrh<br>Neroli (orange blossom)<br>Patchouli<br>Rose<br>Turmeric<br>Vetivert<br>Ylang Ylang |
| **Spikenard** | A tender, flowering herb or plant<br><br>Dried crushed rhizomes and roots<br><br>Valeriancaceae | Woody<br><br>Medium | Very sweet, intense, woody, spicy, animal, valerian root, ginger, cardamom, with tones of fresh-cut grass; becomes less intense and delicately woody, with undertones of spice, fresh pea, and hay, with sweet and tenaciously lingering dry-out notes of fresh pea and hay | Bergamot<br>Cardamom<br>Coriander<br>Ginger<br>Grapefruit<br>Lemon<br>Lime<br>Mandarin<br>Nutmeg<br>Orange bitter<br>Petitgrain | Chamomile Roman<br>Cypress<br>Geranium<br>Lavender<br>Patchouli<br>Pine | Cinnamon leaf<br>Frankincense<br>Myrrh<br>Neroli<br>Rose<br>Turmeric<br>Valerian<br>Vetivert |

| Essential Oil | Plant type | Scent Group — Strength / Intensity | Scent profile | Compatible Essential Oils | | |
|---|---|---|---|---|---|---|
| | | | | Top notes (most volatile, uplifting) | Middle notes (body notes, balancing) | Base notes (tenacious, lingering, grounding) |
| Tea Tree | A shrub or small tree. Leaves, terminal twigs and branches. Myrtaceae | Spicy. Medium | Fresh, strong, citrussy, nutmeg-like, piney, camphoraceous, slightly metallic (yet hints of sweetness), with warm, camphoraceous, medicinal body notes and dry-out notes of weak or little character | Bergamot, Cardamom, Coriander, Cajeput, Eucalyptus, Grapefruit, Lemon, Lime, Lemongrass, Mandarin, Nutmeg, Niaouli, Orange bitter, Peppermint, Petitgrain, Clary Sage | Cypress, Geranium, Lavender, Marjoram, Myrtle, Oregano, Pine, Rosemary | Cinnamon leaf, Clove bud, Myrrh, Rose |
| Thyme | A perennial, low-growing, woody-based or stemmed, evergreen subshrub. Fresh or partially dried leaves and flowering tops. Lamiaceae (Labiatae) | Herbal. High | Red thyme: pungent, phenolic, camphoraceous, medicinal, with warm, resinous, green-herbaceous, spicy-wood body notes and herbaceous-spicy to mild dry-out notes. White thyme: fresh, powerful, thyme-like, herbaceous, camphoraceous, medicinal, phenolic, terpenic, fruity, spicy, with herbaceous-spicy middle notes and mild dry-out notes | Bergamot, Cajeput, Cardamom, Clary Sage, Eucalyptus, Grapefruit, Lemon, Lemongrass, Lime, Mandarin, May Chang, Niaouli, Nutmeg, Orange bitter, Petitgrain | Lavender, Marjoram, Melissa, Oregano, Pine, Rosemary | Cinnamon leaf, Myrrh, Rose |

| | | | | | | | |
|---|---|---|---|---|---|---|---|
| Turmeric | A perennial herbaceous, flowering plant; Chopped rhizomes; Zingiberaceae | Spicy | Medium | Fresh, spicy, spicy-woody, sweet, orange, ginger, rooty, with lingering sweet-earthy, softly spicy body and dry-out notes | Bergamot, Cardamom, Caraway, Coriander, Ginger, Grapefruit, Lemon, Lemongrass, Lime, Mandarin, Nutmeg, Orange bitter, Palmarosa, Petitgrain | Chamomile German, Geranium, Lavender, Black Pepper | Cinnamon leaf, Clove bud, Frankincense, Jasmine, Myrrh, Neroli (orange blossom), Patchouli, Rose, Spikenard, Vetivert, Ylang Ylang |
| Turpentine | A tall erect evergreen tree with a reddish-brown bark, and short stout needle producing branches; Oleoresin gum; Pinaceae | Terpenic | Medium | Warm, fresh, balsam, woody, terpene, sweet, coniferous, piney | Bergamot, Eucalyptus, Grapefruit | Cypress, Juniper Berry, Lavender, Lemon, Rosemary | Cedarwood, Frankincense |
| Valerian | An upright herbaceous plant; Dried, chopped rhizomes; Valerianaceae | Herbal | Medium | Pungent, fresh, green top notes that quickly give way to warm, woody, balsamic, rooty, animal, musky notes, with tenacious base notes sometimes likened to peas or smell socks (the later transcended by its therapeutic value) | Bergamot, Grapefruit, Lemon, Lime, Mandarin, Orange bitter, Petitgrain, Clary Sage | Chamomile(s), Geranium, Lavender, Pine, Rosemary, Yarrow | Cedarwood Atlas, Patchouli, Rose, Spikenard |

| Essential Oil | Plant type | Scent Group Strength / Intensity | Scent profile | Compatible Essential Oils | | |
|---|---|---|---|---|---|---|
| | | | | Top notes (most volatile, uplifting) | Middle notes (body notes, balancing) | Base notes (tenacious, lingering, grounding) |
| Vetivert | Tall grass with brownish–purple flowers<br><br>Dried, chopped roots and rootlets<br><br>Poaceae (Gramineae) | Woody<br><br>Medium | Sweet, earthy, woody top notes, with rich, complex, burnt, smoky, woody, rooty, balsamic, amber body notes that have hints of grapefruit and tenacious woody earth dry-out notes | Bergamot<br>Ginger<br>Grapefruit<br>Juniper berry<br>Lemon<br>Lemongrass<br>Lime<br>Mandarin<br>May Chang<br>Orange bitter<br>Palmarosa<br>Clary Sage | Geranium<br>Lavender<br>Marjoram<br>Melissa<br>Peppermint<br>Yarrow | Cedarwood Atlas<br>Frankincense<br>Jasmine<br>Neroli (orange blossom)<br>Patchouli<br>Rose<br>Sandalwood<br>Spikenard<br>Turmeric<br>Ylang Ylang |
| Yarrow | Upright perennial herb<br><br>Dried herbs<br><br>Asteraceae (Compositae) | Herbal<br><br>High | Fresh, green, sweet (almost sickly), intense, medicinal, phenolic, and fruity, with herbaceous, slightly camphoraceous body notes and warm, hay-like, tobacco-like dry-out notes; very similar to German chamomile | Bergamot<br>Eucalyptus<br>Grapefruit<br>Lemon<br>Lime<br>Mandarin<br>Orange bitter<br>Petitgrain | Chamomile(s)<br>Geranium<br>Helichrysum<br>Juniper berry<br>Lavender<br>Black Pepper<br>Peppermint<br>Pine<br>Rosemary | Cedarwood Atlas<br>Neroli (orange blossom)<br>Rose<br>Valerian<br>Vetivert<br>Ylang Ylang |

| Ylang Ylang | Tall, slim, tropical, evergreen, smooth-barked tree or woody climber<br><br>Freshly picked flowers<br><br>Annonaceae | Floral<br><br>Medium | Strong, sweet, heavy, floral, jasmine, lily, spicy, and medicated notes, with floral, fruity-spicy middle tones, then sweet, balsamic, floral, medicated dry-out notes | Bergamot<br>Caraway<br>Cardamom<br>Coriander<br>Galbanum<br>Ginger<br>Grapefruit<br>Lemon<br>Lemongrass<br>Lime<br>Mandarin<br>May Chang<br>Orange bitter<br>Palmarosa<br>Clary Sage<br>ς | Chaste Tree<br>Frankincense<br>Helichrysum<br>Lavender<br>Marjoram<br>Melissa<br>Myrtle<br>Oregano<br>Black Pepper<br>Petitgrain<br>Yarrow<br><br>*Most woods, florals and fruits* | Cedarwood Atlas<br>Cinnamon leaf<br>Clove bud<br>Jasmine<br>Myrrh<br>Neroli (orange blossom)<br>Patchouli<br>Rose<br>Spikenard<br>Sandalwood<br>Turmeric<br>Vetivert |

# REFERENCES

Redfield, James. *The Celestine Prophecy*. Bantam Books, London (1994).

Wohlleben, Peter. *The Hidden Life of Trees*. William Collins, London. p 15, 16 (2017).

Sheldrake, Merlin (2021) *Entangled Life: How fungi make our worlds, change our minds, and shape our futures.* Vintage, Penguin Random House UK. p 235 (2021).

Bush, Zach. Quorum Sensing. Tree Weaver. *https://treeweaver59.home. blog/2021/05/27/quorum-sensing-by-dr-zach-bush/* (2021)

Bush, Zach. The Year of Connection and Quorum Sensing with Dr. Zach Bush (Clip). *Evolution of Medicine. Interviewer James Maskell https:// www.youtube.com/watch?v=7JqdBiN8opw* (2023). Full Interview: 2023 The Year of Connection. The Critical Nature of Reconnection. *https://goevomed. com/podcasts/the-year-of-connection* (2023).

Tan, Ling, Fei-fei Liao, Lin-zi Long, Xiao-chang Ma, Yu-xuan Peng, Jie-ming Lu, Hua Qu and Chang-geng Fu. Essential oils for treating anxiety: a systematic review of randomised controlled trials and network meta-analysis. *Frontiers in Public Health. https://www.ncbi.nlm.nih.gov/pmc/ articles/PMC10267315/* (2003).

Zsido, Andras N., Szidalisz A. Teleki, Kristina Csokasi, Sandor Rozsa and Szabolcs A. Bandi. Development of the short version of the Spielberger state-trait anxiety inventory. *Psychiatry Research. https://pubmed.ncbi.nlm. nih.gov/32563747/* (2020).

Spielberger, Charles Donald Ph.D. State-Trait Anxiety Inventory for Adults. *American Psychological Association. https://psycnet.apa.org/ doiLanding?doi=10.1037%2Ft06496-000* (1983).

Haig, Matt. *Reasons to Stay Alive*. Cannongate Books, Edinburgh. p 189 (2016).

Aron, Elaine N. *The Highly Sensitive Person: How to thrive when the world overwhelms you.* Thornsons, Harper Collins. p 10 (1999).

Dosari, Mohammed, Saud K. AlDayel, Khalid M. Alduraibi, Abdulaziz A. AlTurki, Fahad Aljehaiman, Sultan Alamri, Hamad S. Alshammari, and Mosad Alsuwilem. Prevalence of Highly Sensitive Personality and its Relationship with Depression, and Anxiety in the Saudi General Population. *Cureus Journal of Medical Science 15 (https://www.ncbi.nlm.nih. gov/pmc/articles/PMC10758235/)* (2023).

Farmer, Antonia S., Todd B. Kashdan. Stress sensitivity and stress generation in social anxiety disorder: a temporal process approach. *Journal of Abnormal Psychology 124(1):102-14 https://pubmed.ncbi.nlm.nih. gov/25668437/* (2015).

Aron, Elaine N. Revisiting Jung's concept of innate sensitivities. *Journal of Analytical Psychology 49(3):337-67 https://pubmed.ncbi.nlm.nih. gov/15149444/* (2004).

Tan, Siang Yong and A. Yip. Hans Seyle (1907-1982): Founder of stress theory. *Singapore Medical Journal 59(4) 170-171. https://www.ncbi.nlm. nih.gov/pmc/articles/PMC5915631/* (2018).

Oxford English Dictionary. *https://www.oed.com/search/dictionary/?scope=Entries&q=stress* (2023).

Haig, Matt. *Reasons to Stay Alive.* Cannongate Books, Edinburgh, p. 189 (2016).

O'Niell, Barbara. *Insomnia.* Sandpoint SDA. Youtube. *https://www.youtube.com/watch?v=p_1qqzywKD8* (2022).

Godfrey, Heather Dawn. *Healing with Essential Oils.* Healing Arts Press, Rochester Vermont. p 141, 165 – 179 (2022).

Heying, Heather and Bret Weinstein. *A Hunter-Gather's Guide to the 21st Century: Evolution and the challenges of modern life.* Swift Press (2022).

Ji, Sayer. Paradise's Farmacy: Herbal Healing and Regenerative Farming Straight from Hawaii. *https://unite.live/greenmedinfo/ greenmedinfo?recording_id=772* (2022).

Ji, Sayer. Regenerate: *Unlocking your body's radical resilience through the new biology.* Hay House (2020).

Wood, Matthew. *Holistic Medicine and the Extracellular Matrix: the science of healing at the cellular level:* Healing Arts Press, Rochester Vermont (2021).

Gagliano, Monica. The minds of plants: Thinking the unthinkable. *Cummunicative and Integrative Biology. Taylor and Francis Group. vol 10 no 2. https://www.researchgate.net/publication/313828053_The_mind_of_plants_Thinking_the_unthinkable.* (2017).

Pollack, Gerald. Water, Cells and Life: The Fourth Phase of Water. *TEDx Talks, New York https://www.youtube.com/watch?v=p9UC0chfXcg* (November 21, 2016).

Pollack, Gerald. Water Isn't What You Think It Is. The Fourth Phase of Water. *Biodiversity for a Livable Climate. https://bio4climate.org/article/water-isnt-what-you-think-it-is-the-fourth-phase-of-water-by-gerald-pollack/* (2019).

Fado, Rut, Anna Molins, Rocio Rojas and Nuria Casals. Feeding the Brain: effect of Nutrients on Cognition, Synaptic Function, and AMPA Receptors. *Journal of Nutrients 14(19):4137. https://www.ncbi.nlm.nih.gov/pmc/articles/PMC9572450/* (2022).

Larrieu, Thomas and Sophie Lave. Food for Mood: Relevance of Nutritional Omega-3 Fatty Acids for Depression and Anxiety. *Frontiers in Psychology 9:1047. https://www.ncbi.nlm.nih.gov/pmc/articles/PMC6087749/* (2018).

Chang, Chia-Yu, Der-Shin Ke and Jen-Yin Chen. Essential fatty acids and human brain. *Act Neurological Taiwanica 18(4):231–41. https://pubmed.ncbi.nlm.nih.gov/20329590/* (2009).

Bourre, J. M. Effects of nutrients (in food) on the structure and function of the nervous system: update on dietary requirements for brain. Part 1: micronutrients. *The Journal of Nutrition, Health, and Aging 10(5):377-85 https://pubmed.ncbi.nlm.nih.gov/17066209/* (2006).

Heying, Heather and Bret Weinstein. *A Hunter-Gather's Guide to the 21st Century: Evolution and the challenges of modern life.* Swift Press (2022).

Mahindru, Aditya, Pradeep Patil and Varun Agrawal. Role of Physical

Activity on Mental Health and Well-Being: A review. *Cureus ed. 33475: 15(1). https://www.ncbi.nlm.nih.gov/pmc/articles/PMC9902068/* (2023).

Mikkelsen, Kathleen, Lily Stojanovska, Momir Polenakovic, Marijan Bosevski and Vasso Aposstolopoulos. Exercise and mental health. *MATURITAS: An international journal of midlife health and beyond, vol 106: 48-56. https://www.maturitas.org/article/S0378-5122(17)30856-3/fulltext* (2017).

Oschman, James L., Gaetan Chevalier and Richard Brown. The effects of grounding (earthing) on inflammation, the immune response, wound healing, and prevention and treatment of chronic inflammatory and autoimmune diseases. *Journal of Inflammation Research, 8: 83-96. https://www.ncbi.nlm.nih.gov/pmc/articles/PMC4378297/* (2015).

Chevalier, Gaetan, Stephen T. Sinatra, James L. Oschman, Darol Sokal and Pawel Sokal. Earthing: health Implications of Reconnecting the Human Body to the Earth's Surface Electrons. *Journal of Environmental and Public Health, 291541. https://www.ncbi.nlm.nih.gov/pmc/articles/PMC3265077/* (2012).

Peterson, Jordan. This is What Happens When You're Bored. *Success Now. You Tube. https://www.youtube.com/watch?v=DUOO9Uum3ZM (2023)* (sourced 3rd February 2024).

Rawat, Prem. *Hear Yourself: How to find peace in noisy world.* Harper One, New York, (2021).

Tolle, Eckhart. *Stillness Speaks: A Guide to Spiritual Enlightenment.* Yellow Kite Books, London, (2023).

Paver, Michelle. *Vipers Daughter.* Zephyr, Heads of Zues, London (2020).

Godfrey, Heather Dawn. *Essential Oils for the Whole Body.* Healing Arts Press, Rochester Vermont. p 171 -173 (2019).

Munir, Sadaf, Sasidhar Gunturu, Muhammad Abbas. Seasonal Affective Disorder. *StatPearls Publishing. Treasure Island, Florida USA. https://pubmed.ncbi.nlm.nih.gov/33760504/* (2024).

De Vaus, June, Matthew J. Hornesy, Peter Kuppens and Brock Bastian.

Exploring the East-West Divide in Prevalence of Affective Disorder: A Case for Cultural Differences in Coping with Negative Emotion. *Personality and Social Psychology Review, vol. 22 issue 3, Sage Journals. https://journals.sagepub.com/doi/full/10.1177/1088868317736222* (2017).

Rosen, L. N., S. D. Targum, M. Terman, M. J. Bryant, H. Hoffman, S. F. Kasper, J. R. Hamovit, J. P. Docherty, B. Welch and N. E. Rosenthal. Prevalence of seasonal affective disorder at four latitudes. *Psychiatry Research, 31(2):131-44. National Centre for Biotechnology Information. https://pubmed.ncbi.nlm.nih.gov/2326393/* (1990).

Kuehner, Christine. Why is depression more common among women than men? *The Lancet Psychiatry 4(2):146-158. https://pubmed.ncbi.nlm.nih.gov/27856392/* (2017).

Chotai, Jayanti, Kristina Smedh, Carolina Johansson, Lars-Goran Nilsson and Rolf Adolfsson. An epidemiological study on gender differences in self-reported seasonal changes in mood and behaviour in a general population of northern Sweden. *Nordic Journal of Psychiatry 58(6):429-37. https://pubmed.ncbi.nlm.nih.gov/16195086/#:~:text=SAD%20was%20found%20in%202.2,with%20age%20in%20both%20genders* (2004)

Farmer, Antonina S. and Todd B. Kashdan. Stress sensitivity and stress generation in social anxiety disorder: a temporal process approach. *Journal of Abnormal Psychology 124(1):102-14. https://pubmed.ncbi.nlm.nih.gov/25688437/* (2015).

Godfrey, Heather Dawn. *Essential Oils for Mindfulness and Meditation.* Healing Arts Press, Rochester, Vermont USA. p 126-127 (2019).

Godfrey, Heather Dawn. *Essential Oils for the Whole Body: The dynamics of topical application and Absorption.* Healing Arts Press, Rochester, Vermont USA. p 155 – 176 (2020).

Sowndhararajan, Kandasamy, and Songmin Kim. Influence of Fragrance on Human Psychophysiological Activity: With special reference to human electroencephalographic response. *Scientia Pharmaceutica, National Library of Medicine. 84(4): 724-752* (2016).

Soto-Vasjuez, Marilu Roxana, and Paul Alan Arkin Alvarado-

Garcia. Aromatherapy with two essential oils from Satureja genre and mindfulness meditation to reduce anxiety in humans. *Journal of Traditional and Complementary Medicine 7(1)   https://www.researchgate. net/publication/304536506_Aromatherapy_with_two_essential_oils_from_ Satureja_genre_and_mindfulness_meditation_to_reduce_anxiety_in_humans* (2016).

Santos, Everton Renan Quaresma dos, Jose Guilherme S. Maia, Eneas Andrade Fontes-Junior, Christiane do-Socorro and Ferraz Maia. Linalool as a Therapeutic and Medicinal Tool in Depression Treatment: A Review. *Current Neuropharmacology, Bentham Science Publishers, 20(6): 1073-1092. https://www.ncbi.nlm.nih.gov/pmc/articles/PMC9886818/* (2022).

Tan, Ling, Fei-fei Liao, Lin-zi Long, Xiao-chang Ma, Yu-xuan Peng, Jie-ming Lu, Hua Qu and Chang-geng Fu (2023) Essential oils for treating anxiety: a systematic review of randomised controlled trials and network meta-analysis. *Frontiers in Public Health. https://www.ncbi.nlm.nih.gov/ pmc/articles/PMC10267315/* (2023).

Seo, Eunhye, Yoonan Cho, Jeong-Min Lee and Geun Hee Seol. Inhalation of Pelargonium graveolens Essential Oil Alleviates Pain and related Anxiety and Stress in Patients with Lumber Spinal Stenosis and Moderate to Severe Pain. *Pharmaceuticals (Basel). https://pubmed.ncbi.nlm.nih. gov/38275987/* (2023).

Ozer, Zulfinaz, Neslihan Teke, Gulcan Bahcecioglu Turan and Ayse Nefise Bahcecik. Effectiveness of lemon essential oil in reducing test anxiety in nursing student. *Explore New York, Elsevier. https://pubmed.ncbi.nlm.nih. gov/35190270/* (2022).

Alvarado-Garcia, Paul Alen Arkin, Marilu Roxana Soto-Vasquez, Luis Enrique Rosaes-Cerquin, Bertha Mirella Alfaro-Ttito and Elda Maritza Rodrigo-Villanueva. Anxiolytic Effect of Essential Oils Extracted from Lippia alba and Lippia citriodora. *Pharmacognosy Journal 13, 6, 1377-1383. https://www.phcogj.com/article/1672* (2021).

Sherzadegan, Razieh, Mohammad Gholami, Shirin Hasanvand, Mehdi Birjandi and Afsaneh Beiranvand. Effects of geranium aroma on anxiety among patients with acute myocardial infarction: A triple-blind randomised clinical trial. *Complementary Therapies in Clinical Practice p 201-206. https://pubmed.ncbi.nlm.nih.gov/29122262/* (2017).

Zhang, Nan, Jie Chen, Wenyan Dong and Lei Yao. The Effect of Copaiba Oil Odor on Anxiety Relief in Adults under Mental Workload: A Randomised Controlled Trial. *Evidence Based Complementary and Alternative Medicine. https://pubmed.ncbi.nlm.nih.gov/35449818/* (2022).

Jia, Yanzhou, Yao Wang, Xiaofei Zhang, Yajun Shi, Yulin Liang, Dongyan Guo and Ming Yang. Action mechanism of roman chamomile in the treatment of anxiety disorder based on network pharmacology. *Journal of Food Biochemistry 45(1). https://pubmed.ncbi.nlm.nih.gov/33152801/* (2021).

Shrivastava, Janmejai K., Eswar Shankar and Sanjay Gupta. Chamomile: A herbal medicine of the past with bright future. *Molecular Medicine Report, vol 3 issue 6 p 895-901. https://www.ncbi.nlm.nih.gov/pmc/articles/PMC2995283/* (2011).

Achour, Miriam, Intidhar Ben Salem, Farhana Ferdousi, Menel Nouira, Maha Ben Fredj, Ali Mtiraoui, Hiroko Isoda and Saad Saguem. Rosemary Tea Consumption Alters Peripheral Anxiety and Depression Biomarkers: A Pilot Study in Limited Healthy Volunteers. *Journal of the American Nutrition Association 41(3): 240-249. https://pubmed.ncbi.nlm.nih.gov/33565922/* (2022).

Ferlemi, Anastasia-Varvara, Antigoni Katsikoudi, Vassiliki G. Kontogeianne, Tahsin F. Kellici, Grigoris Iatrou, Fontini N. Lamari, Andreas G. Tzakos and Marigoula Margarity. Rosemary tea consumption results to anxiolytic- and anti-depressant-like behaviour of adult male mice and inhibits all cerebral area and liver cholinesterase activity; phytochemical investigation and in silico studies. *Chemico-Biological Interactions 237: 47-57. https://pubmed.ncbi.nlm.nih.gov/25910439/* (2015).

Bazrafshan, Mohammad-Rafi, Mozhgan Jokar, Nasrin Shakrpour and Hamed Delam. The effect of lavender herbal tea on the anxiety and depression of the elderly: A randomised clinical trial. *Complementary Therapies in Medicine vol 50. Elsevier. https://www.sciencedirect.com/science/article/abs/pii/S0965229919316292* (2020).

Ghazizadeh, Javid Saeed, Sadigh-Eteghad, Wolfgang Marx, Ali Fakhari, Sanex Hamedeyazdan, Mohammadali Torbati, Somalyeh Taheri-Tarighi, Mostafa Araj-Khodael and Majgan Mirghafourvand (2021) The effects of lemon balm (Melissa officinalis L.) on depression and anxiety in clinical trials: A systematic review and meta-analysis. *Phytotherapy Research 35(12): 6690-6705. https://pubmed.ncbi.nlm.nih.gov/34449930/* (2021).

Vasey, Christopher N. D. *The Acid-Alkaline Diet for Optimum Health: Restore your health by creating pH balance in your diet.* Healing Arts Press, Vermont USA (2018).

Sattayakhom, Apsorn, Sineewanlaya Wichit and Phanit Koomhin. The Effects of Essential Oils on the Nervous System: A Scoping Review. *Molecules (Basal, Switzerland) 28(9): 3771. https://pubmed.ncbi.nlm.nih. gov/37175176/* (2023).

Kennedy, Emma, Claire L. Niedzwidz. The association of anxiety and stress-related disorders the C-reactive protein (CRP) within UK Biobank. *Brain, Behaviour and Immunity, Elsevier. https://www.ncbi.nlm.nih.gov/ pmc/articles/PMC8741412/* (2022)

Ravi, Meghna, Andrew H. Miller and Vasiliki Michopoulos. The Immunology of Stress and the Impact of Inflammation on the Brain and Behaviour. *BJPsych Adv. (Suppl 3): 158-165. https://www.ncbi.nlm.nih.gov/ pmc/articles/PMC8158089/* (2012).

Michopoulos, Vasiliki, Abigail Powers, Charles F. Gillespie, Kerry J. Ressier and Tanja Jovanovic. Inflammation in Fear-and Anxiety-Based Disorders: PTSD, GAD, and Beyond. *Neuropsychopharmacology 21(1): 254-270. https://www.ncbi.nlm.nih.gov/pmc/articles/PMC5143487/* (2017).

Vogelzans, N., A. T. F. Beekman, P. de Jongs and B>W. J. H. Phenninx. Anxiety disorders and inflammation in a large adult cohort. *Nature, Translational Psychiatry 3(249). https://www.nature.com/articles/tp201327* (2013).

Caro, Daneiva C., David E. Rivera, Yanet Ocampo, Luis A. Franco and Ruben D. Salas Pharmacological evaluation of *Menthis spicata L.* and *Plantago major L.*, Medicinal Plants used to Treat Anxiety and

Insomnia in Colombian Caribbean Coast. *Evidence Based Complementary and Alternative Medicine. https://www.ncbi.nlm.nih.gov/pmc/articles/ PMC6106973/* (2018).

Bensouilah, Janetta, and Philippa Buck. *Aromadermatology: Aromatherapy in the treatment and care of common skin conditions.* Radcliffe Publishing. P 75 – 76 (2006).

Cui, Jieqiong, Meng Li, Yuanyuan Wei, Huayan Li, Xiying He, Qi yang, Zhengkun Li, Jinfeng Duan, Zhao Wu, Qian Chen, Bojun Chen, Gang Li, Xi Ming, Lei Xiong and Dongdong Qin. Inhalation Aromatherapy via Brain-Targeted Nasal Delivery: Natural Volatiles or Essential Oils on Mood Disorders. *Frontiers in Pharmacology, 13: 860043. https://www.ncbi. nlm.nih.gov/pmc/articles/pmid/35496310/* (2022).

Soares, Giselle A. Borges, Tanima Bhattacharya, Tulika Chakrabarti, Priti Tagde and Simona Cavalu. Exploring Pharmacological Mechanisms of Essential Oils on the Central Nervous System. *Plants (Basel) 11(1): 21. https://www.ncbi.nlm.nih.gov/pmc/articles/PMC8747111/* (2022).

Fung, Timothy K. H., Benson W. M. Lau, Shirley P. C. Ngai and Hector W. H. Tsang. Therapeutic Effect and Mechanisms of Essential Oils in Mood Disorders: Interaction between the Nervous and respiratory Systems. *International Journal of Molecular Science, 22(9): 4844. https:// www.ncbi.nlm.nih.gov/pmc/articles/PMC8125361/* (2021).

Wu, Xue Shen, Tian Xie, Jing Lin, Hai Zhu Fan, Hong Jiao Huang-Fu, Li Feng Ni, Hui Fang Yan. An investigation of the ability of elemene to pass through the blood-brain barrier and its effect on the brain carcinomas. *The Journal of Pharmacy and Pharmacology 61(12). https://pubmed.ncbi.nlm.nih. gov/19958588/* (2009).

Gallagher, James, Rachael Buchanan and Victoria Gill (2014) Body Clock: What makes you tick. *BBC News. https://www.bbc.co.uk/news/ health-27161671* (2014).

Star-Wolf, Linda, and Anna Cariad-Barrett. *Sacred Medicine of Bee, Butterfly, Earthworm, and Spider: Shamanic teachers of the Instar Medicine Wheel.* Bear and Company, Rochester Vermont USA (2013).

The Good Scents Company. *http://www.thegoodscentscompany.com/essentlx. html* (2025)

# BIBLIOGRAPHY

Ahmadi, Tayebeh, Leila Shabani and Mohammad R. Sabzalian. LED light sources improved the essential oil components and antioxidant activity of two genotypes of lemon balm (Melissa officinalis). *Botanical Studies 62 article no. 9. https://as-botanicalstudies.springeropen.com/articles/10.1186/ s40529-021-00316-7* (2021).

Burr, Chandler. *The Emperor of Scent: A Story of Perfume, Obsession and the Last Mystery of the Senses.* Arrow Books, Penguin Random House, London (2022).

Elshafie, Hazam S., and Ippolito Camele. An Overview of the Biological Effects of Some Mediterranean Essential Oils on Human Health. *Biomedical Research International. https://www.ncbi.nlm.nih.gov/pmc/ articles/PMC5694587/* (2017).

Farhud, Dariush, and Zahra Aryan. Circadian Rhythm, Lifestyle and Health: A Narrative Review. *Iran Journal of Public Health 47(8) 1068-1076. https://www.ncbi.nlm.nih.gov/pmc/articles/PMC6123576/* (2018).

Fung, Timothy K. H., Benson W. M. Lau, Shirley P. C. Ngai and Hector W. H. Tsang. Therapeutic Effect and Mechanisms of Essential Oils in Mood Disorders: Interaction Between Nervous and Respiratory System. *International Journal of Molecular Science 22(9): 4844. https://www.ncbi. nlm.nih.gov/pmc/articles/PMC8125361/* (2021).

Ghazizadeh, Javid, Saeed Sadkigh-Eteghad, Wolfgang Marx, Ali Fakhori, Sanaz Hamedeyazdan, Mohmmadali Torbati, Solaiyeh Taheri-Tarighi, Mostafa Araj-Khodaei and Mojgan Mirghafourvand. The effects of lemon balm (Melissa officinalis L.) on depression and anxiety in clinical trials: A systematic review and meta-analysis. *Phytotherapy Research 35(12): 6690-6705. https://pubmed.ncbi.nlm.nih.gov/34449930/* (2021).

Gooley, Tristan. *Wild Signs and Star Paths: 52 keys that will open your eyes, ears and mind to the world around you.* Sceptre, Hodder and Stoughton, London (2018).

Hwang, Jin He. The Effects of the Inhalation Method using Essential Oils on Blood Pressure and Stress of Clients with Essential Hypertension. *Journal of Korean Academy of Nursing vol 36(7). https://www.jkan.or.kr/DOIx.php?id=10.4040/jkan.2006.36.7.1123* (2006).

Jia, Yanzhou, Junbo Zou, Yao Wang, Xiaofei Zhang, Yajun Shi, Yulin Liang, Dongyan Guo and Ming Yang. Action mechanisms of roman chamomile in the treatment of anxiety disorder based on network pharmacology. *Journal of Food Biochemistry 45(1). https://pubmed.ncbi.nlm.nih.gov/33152801/* (2012).

Karadag, Ezgi, Sevgin Samancioglu, Dilek Ozden and Ercan Bakir. Effects of aromatherapy on sleep quality and anxiety of patients. *Nursing in Critical Care 22(2): 105-112. https://onlinelibrary.wiley.com/toc/14785153/2017/22/2* (2017).

Kennedy, David O., Wendy Little, Crystal F. Haskell and Andrew B Scholey. Melissa officinalis Valeriana officinalis have an anti-anxiety effect during laboratory-induced stress. *Phytotherapy Research 20(2): 96-102. https://pubmed.ncbi.nlm.nih.gov/16444660/* (2006).

Kritkakusky, Randy. *Without Reservation: Awakening to Native American Spirituality and the Ways of our Ancestors.* Bear and Company, Rochester Vermont, (2020).

Leon, Michael and Cynthia Woo. Environment Enrichment and Successful Aging. *Frontiers in Behavioural Neuroscience vol 12. https://www.frontiersin.org/articles/10.3389/fnbeh.2018.00155/full* (2018).

Leon, Michael and Cynthia Woo. Olfactory loss is a predisposing factor for depression, while olfactory enrichment is an effective treatment for depression. *Frontiers in Neuroscience vol 16. https://www.frontiersin.org/articles/10.3389/fnins.2022.1013363/full* (2022).

Lima, Vandimilli A., Fernanda V. Pacheco, Rafaella P. Avelar, Ivan C. A. Alvarenga, Jose Eduardo B. P. Pinto and Amauri A. de Alvarenga. Growth, photosynethetic pigments and production of essential oil of long-pepper under different light conditions. *Agrarian Sciences, Anais da Academia Brasileira de Ciencias 89(02). https://www.scielo.br/j/aabc/a/xZcgGNHT7s7gKPvSXRYtxpm/?lang=en* (2017).

Lovelock, James Lovelock. *GAIA.* Oxford University Press. (2016).

Maury, Marguerite Maury. *The Secret of Life and Youth.* The C.W. Daniel Company Limited, Saffron Walden. p 80-81 (1995).

May, Kathrine. *Wintering: The power of rest and retreat in difficult times.* Penguin Ryder House, London. (2020).

Meacham, Elizabeth E. PhD. *Earth Spirit Dreaming: Shamanic Ecotherapy Practices.* Findhorn Press, Rochester Vermont (2020).

Milenkovic, Lidija, Zoran S. Ilic, Ljubomir Sunic, Nadica Tmusic, Ljiljana Stanjevic and Dragan Cvetkovic. Modification of light intensity influence essential oils content, composition and antioxidant activity of thyme, marjoram and oregano. *Saudi Journal of Biological Sciences. Vol 28 Issue 11. https://www.sciencedirect.com/science/article/pii/S1319562X2100591X* (2021).

Misra, Pooja, Deepamala Maji, Ashutosh Awasthi, Shiv Shanker Pandey, Anju Yadav, Alok Pandey, Dharmedra Saika, C. S. Vivek Babu and Alok Kalra. Vulnerability of Soil Microbiome to Monocropping of Medicinal and Aromatic Plants and its Restoration Through Intercropping and Organic Amendments. *Frontiers in Microbiology. https://www.frontiersin. org/articles/10.3389/fmicb.2019.02604/full* (2019).

Peterson, Jordan. *12 Rules for Life: An Antidote to Chaos.* Penguin Books, UK. (2019).

Peterson, Jordan. Advice for People with Depression. *Motivation Ark, You Tube. https://www.youtube.com/watch?v=2e5a1TIl_Ts* (2022). (sourced 31st January 2024)

Peterson, Jordan. *Beyond Order: 12 More Rules for Life.* Penguin Books, UK (2021).

Peterson, Jordan. The Horrific Truth About Depression That Everyone Must Know. *The Motive, You Tube (sourced 31st January 2024). https:// www.youtube.com/watch?v=2e5a1TIl_Ts* (2023).

Ramos, Ygor Jesse, Claudete da Costa-Oliveira, Irene Candido-Fonseca, George Azevedo de Queiroz, Elsie Frankilin Guimaraes, Anna C. Antunes E Defaveri, Nicholas John Sadgrove and Davyson de Lima Moreira.

Advanced Chemophenetic Analysis of essential Oil from Leaves of *Piper gaudichaudianum* Kunth (Piperaceae) Using a New Reduction-Oxidisation Index to Explore Seasonal and Circadian Rhythms. *Plants (Basel), National Library of Medicine. 10(10):2116 https://pubmed.ncbi.nlm.nih. gov/34685925/#:~:text=Chemical%20analysis%20demonstrated%20that%20 the,giving%20a%20total%20of%2019* (2021).

Ribeiro, Aurislaine S., Mariana S. Ribeiro, Suzan K. V. Bertolucci, Wanderley J. M. Bittencourt, Alexandre A. de Carvalho, Wesley N. Tostes, Eduardo Alves and Jose E. B. P. Pinto. Colored shade nets indued changes in growth, anatomy and essential oil of Pogostemon cablin. *Annals of Brazilian Academy of Sciences 90(2): 1823-1835 https://pdfs.semanticscholar. org/68a0/8e19f192377c76731b4ddb8f5e14d07820ea.pdf* (2018).

Schoffro Cook, Michelle. *Super-Powered Immunity Starts in the Gut.* Healing Arts Press, Rochester Vermont (2024).

Setzer, William N. Essential oils and anxiolytic aromatherapy. Sage Journals. *https://journals.sagepub.com/doi/ abs/10.1177/1934578X0900400928* (2009).

Silva, Sebastiao G., Pablo Luis B. Figueiredo, Lidiane D. Nascimento, Wanessa A. da Costa, Jose Guilherme S. Maia and Eloisa Helena A. Andrade (2018) Planting and seasonal and circadian evaluation of the thymol-type oil from *lippa thymoides* Mart. Schauer. *Chemical Central Journal 12, article no: 113. https://bmcchem.biomedcentral.com/ articles/10.1186/s13065-018-0484-4* (2018).

Srivastava, Janmejai K., Eswar Shankar and Sanjay Gupta. Chamomile: A herbal medicine of the past with bright future. *Molecular Medicine Reports 3(6): 895-901. https://www.ncbi.nlm.nih.gov/pmc/articles/PMC2995283/* (2010).

Tisserand, Robert and Rodney Young. *Essential Oil Safety 2nd ed.* Churchill Livingstone, Edinburgh. P 387, 292-293 (2014).

Willem, Jean-Peirre. *Alzheimer's. Aromatherapy, and the Sense of Smell: Essential Oils to Prevent Cognitive Loss and Restore Memory.* Healing Arts Press, Rochester, Vermont (2021).

Yool, Lee, Jeffrey M. Field and Amita Segal. Circadian Rhythms, Disease and Chronotherapy. *Journal of Biological Rhythms vol 36 issue 6. https:// journals.sagepub.com/doi/full/10.1177/07487304211044301* (2021).

Zheng, Xuehan, Kun Zhang, Yanbin Zhao and Karl Fent. Environmental chemical affect circadian rhythms: An under-explored effect influence health and fitness in animal and humans. *Environment International, Elsevier vol 149. https://www.sciencedirect.com/scien* (2021).

# NOTES